THE FOUNTAIN OF YOU

LiFe should
always be
FUN -
Rick

*Scan this QR Code
to learn more about
this title*

Cover and interior design by Emily Coats
Water Splash © Jay_cz. Bigstockphoto.com
Training © Unsplash. Pixabay.com
Fountain © Hans. Pixabay.com
Senior Man Lifting Large Weights © Waxart. Dreamstime.com
Man with muscles © Geotrac. Dreamstime.com
Boy with dumbbells © Denys Prokofyev. Dreamstime.com

* R.A. Freedman is accredited by the International Sports Sciences Association

Publisher: Inkwater Press

Paperback
ISBN-13 978-1-62901-279-7 | ISBN-10 1-62901-279-3

Printed in the U.S.A.
All paper is acid free and meets all ANSI standards for archival quality paper.

3 5 7 9 10 8 6 4 2

THE FOUNTAIN OF YOU

GETTING STRONGER. LIVING LONGER.

Key strategies on fitness and weight management
for a healthier, more vibrant and energetic life

Including the DGOLF Diet Plan

BY CERTIFIED MASTER FITNESS TRAINER*
Richard A. Freedman

Portland•Oregon
inkwaterpress.com

CONTENTS

The secret of change is to focus all your energy, not on fighting the old, but on building the new.

— *Socrates*

FOREWORD

When it comes to healthful living, the vast and growing amount of information we are bombarded with is confusing and daunting. What is important to know about our aging bodies? How important is exercise? What kind of exercise is best? How should we eat? What should we eat? Is mindfulness really important? How much sleep do we need? Is it too late to make a change?

Fifteen years ago Rich Freedman was an overweight, out of shape business executive retiring from a stressful work environment in the corporate energy sector. He began his journey to health, and a second lease on life, when he sought to answer these questions we all ask. In his case, Rich was motivated to live longer than his own father who suffered from both heart disease and lung cancer. We all feel our mortality at some point.

Today Rich is a very knowledgeable Certified Master Fitness Trainer who has distilled his approach to exercise, eating, and living well. He was not born to be a trainer, but rather made himself a great trainer through hard work. He is now sharing his learning with us. The essential thing Rich teaches in this book is that it is not too late! Rich is also a guy who not only talks the talk, but walks the walk.

He explains the latest research and approaches in easy to understand language that will leave anyone, young or older, feeling empowered to begin and travel their own path to healthful living.

Loren E. Jenkins, MD
Orthopaedic Surgery
Portland, Oregon

ACKNOWLEDGMENTS

Human interaction is much like Forrest Gump described, "ya never know what you're going to get." This especially pertains to good ideas. I am fortunate not only to have been provided an education and insights from professionals and colleagues, but from everyday people of all walks of life—people I've met in the gym, people on planes, in shopping malls and from virtually every vocation you can think of including bartenders, maids, lawyers, mail carriers, professors, dentists, doctors, construction workers, and others who were just happy to talk about their approach to staying fit.

My biggest thanks, however, must go to my wife, Linda, who provides me with daily inspiration. I doubt I could have written a word without her encouragement. To my colleague and business partner, PGA Professional Quincy Heard, a big thanks for sharing his great knowledge of the game of golf and his approach to problem solving and performance improvement. I must also acknowledge the fine education I have received from the International Sports Sciences Association (ISSA) of Carpinteria, California. They not only provide fitness certifications, but the educational support services that allow trainers like me to continuously learn and improve. A special thanks also goes to my friend and neighbor, Vicky Kieffer, who helped so much with the photographic illustrations.

I am most grateful for two amazing physicians who reviewed my material and provided their professional knowledge and insight. To Dr. Yuval Raizen of Houston, Texas my utmost appreciation for his expertise and taking the time to review my work, and to Dr. Loren Jenkins of Portland, Oregon who has also been so gracious providing his time, expertise and wisdom. If you happen to be a patient of either of these two fine physicians, you are in the best of care.

PREFACE

THE FATHER TIME SYNDROME

You wake up in the morning and after your cup of java you feel ready to face the day. The next day you wake up and feel pretty much the same as the day before. Pretty soon, you're trapped in what we shall call the "Father Time" Syndrome—the belief that how you feel each day is pretty much how you're going to feel the next day.

You have every reason to believe your body will behave just as it has in the past. The flaw in this logic is simple—things are going to change. Arthritis, diabetes, heart disease and cancer generally take years to show their ugly heads and when they do the outcomes can be catastrophic. The long term effects of obesity, smoking, lack of exercise and poor nutritional choices are well known. It's just that more often than not these calamities do not translate into lifestyle changes until it's too late. Much of the hoopla around health care insurance seems to be focused on what happens after you need medical attention, but what about preventive care?

A recent visit to a friend's house opened my already wide eyes to the reality that only 35 percent of the adult American population is classified as having a normal weight.[1] The trend to poor dietary habits and sedentary lifestyles has created a devastating epidemic of weight gain and the costly health issues that come with it.

My entrance to this home revealed most of the problem in plain sight: candy, pies, cookies, cakes, potato chips, chocolate, soda, cereals with added sugar, syrups, fruit juices and more. All of these "foods" contain high amounts of sodium, saturated fat or sugar, not to mention the calories. What's really wrong with the ingredients of these everyday foods so many people eat? After all, our bodies run on sugar molecules (glycogen) and sodium is an important electrolyte. Fat is also needed in our diet for proper cellular function. The answer is the same as what's wrong with too much water—you can drown in it. It's not that indulging in limited amounts of these tasty treats would be so harmful. It's the cumulative effect that produces slower metabolisms, weight gain and the diseases that come with it.

As a fitness trainer I see many clients who have not only over-indulged, but who have also led a sedentary lifestyle. This duo can cause disease, bodily decay and premature aging. The effects of such poor choices are in many cases reversible, unless it's too late. Hopefully, I caught you in the nick of time.

EMBRACING THE HUMAN CONDITION

The large mass of aggregated neurons inside your head is responsible for an amazing physiological mixture of consciousness and self-awareness. This is what separates us from the rest of the animal kingdom. Our ability to understand the concept of time and space, to think, to reason and create gives us almost limitless potential to master our universe. We have developed amazing technologies, civilizations, and culture all of which are the result of individual and collective achievement. We have delved into the world of sub-atomic particles, quantum mechanics, biochemistry and the elements that comprise our universe. With such scientific technology and brain power at our disposal, however, it is hard to understand why we often find it so difficult to control the health and wellness of the body sitting just below our amazing brain.

Not long ago I was training at a local gym and came across a man who I guessed to be in his mid 70s working up a substantial sweat on the elliptical trainer next to me. As he dismounted the machine I casually said, "Nice workout, you expended some serious energy!" His lyrical response was as unexpected as it was descriptive. He replied, "I am just a man with a cup sailing in a small boat with a hole in the bottom on an endless sea."

It struck me immediately his metaphor for the importance of caring for his body was spot on. Human beings were created to toil, hunt, chase, climb, farm, protect their young, and if necessary bail water to survive. It should come as no surprise our bodies were not created to sit endlessly in front of an electronic box eating popcorn and drinking flavored carbonated water.

The social, technological, and economic developments of the last century have given us an easy exit from the toils of the past. Work has transformed. While many still labor in the fields, millions of others have discovered the benefits of living in cities and urban areas embracing the technological umbrella that has virtually eliminated the physical effort once required to survive. The problem is our genetics haven't quite adapted to it.

Heart disease, diabetes, arthritis, osteoporosis, some forms of cancer and muscular frailty are more often than not related to a sedentary lifestyle. These conditions have become a "pandemic" our ancestors could not have foreseen.

If we were a mechanical entity, like an automobile, the fix might be easier. Our vehicles come conveniently with specific service instructions. If we do happen to have unscheduled mechanical breakdowns there are thousands of dealerships, repair shops, and auto specialists located in every city and town and there may come a time when a mechanic tells you your vehicle is kaput. The repairs are so expensive or your car is so old parts may not be available. Sound familiar?

Now, consider the human body—not only a mechanical device but a flesh and bone biological wonder. The similarities between your car's operating system and the human body are more than remarkable. The electromechanical automobile was either consciously or subconsciously designed in our likeness and virtually all its operating systems have a close human corollary as illustrated below:

HUMAN SYSTEM	AUTOMOTIVE SYSTEM
Digestive	Fuel system
Respiratory	Air intake
Cardiovascular	Fuel Injection/ carburetor
Muscular	Hydraulics, springs, shock absorbers
Skeletal	Body Frame
Nervous	Electrical system/computer
Lymphatic	Cooling system & misc. filters
Endocrine	Oil, transmission & brake fluid, etc.
Integumentary (skin)	Paint & undercoating
Urinary	Exhaust system
Reproductive	Factory

Comparison of Human and Automotive operating systems

While the human/automobile correlations are certainly not precise there is nevertheless systemic logic in this illustration. The human "machine" processes fuel (carbohydrates, proteins & fats) to create biomechanical energy. An automobile creates electromechanical energy using a variety of fuel options: hydrocarbons, chemical reactive (as in batteries) and several other methods currently under development (e.g. hydrogen). We know it takes routine maintenance to keep our vehicles running properly and it is no different with humans. Just like cars we have our own repair and maintenance shops (doctors, hospitals, clinics, fitness centers, etc).

We know exactly what we need to do to maintain our car. The manufacturers provide a manual and a routine service checklist. Pretty convenient isn't it? Unfortunately, we aren't born with an instructional manual, so how do we maintain our bodies? Can we stay healthy, fit and vibrant as we age? Can we retard or even reverse the aging process? What are the best fuels (foods) for us? How much and what kinds of exercise do we need? Are there ways to reduce the risk of breakdowns (in the form of cancer, heart disease, arthritis, diabetes, osteoporosis, etc)? What about inherited diseases or congenital defects?

Think of the possible answers to the above questions in this way. Suppose you had a broken radiator hose or a loose door hinge. Likely you would look for a mechanic or perhaps a tool to fix the problem. You'd want the solution to be easy, reasonably priced and if there were any instructions, easy to understand. The pages ahead contain just that—the basic instructions and tools to do something really amazing: improve the chance for a longer, healthier and more vibrant life.

Since our health is something we all cherish, we know in its absence it can be difficult to pursue even the most basic activities of daily life. Just about everyone wants to live to a ripe old age and be healthy enough to enjoy the "golden years." Social Security Mortality tables indicate the average American male retiring at age 65 has only a 40 percent chance of living to age 85 and females a bit more at 53 percent. If these same individuals are 25 percent healthier than average, however, these statistics improve to 50 percent for males and 62 percent for females.[2]

A word to the wise before examining the specifics on achieving a healthier and more vibrant life. It is not recommended you begin any program of physical activity or dietary change until you have been medically evaluated by a physician to ensure you understand all the physical risks and you are aware of the facts about engaging in a workout regimen and/or changing your nutrition. Certain medical conditions may increase the risk of injury or fatality. Strength training and aerobic routines raise your blood pressure and heart rate. It would be highly unusual for a physician to recommend you shouldn't exercise or switch to a better diet, but precautions may be necessary. Your medical provider should be the first and best place to start.

Please also note this book has no fine print. There are no hidden caveats as you might see on the bottom of your TV screen in many fitness and diet infomercials. Often these marketing advertisements say "results not typical" or "results achieved only when combined with our diet and exercise plan." The structure here is simple: where physical effort or caloric restriction is required to achieve a given result it won't be hidden down at the bottom of the page in the hope you won't be able to read it. In fact, let's begin with something you should already know; health and fitness require specific modes of exercise for your muscles and metabolism with a diet having the proper macro and micronutrients. It would seem this should be common knowledge, but unfortunately, I have found this to not always be the case.

CHAPTER 1

THE BASIC ELEMENT OF GOOD HEALTH: LIFESTYLE

Medical science has come a long way in the past century. Diseases and chronic conditions which were once a death sentence are now easily controlled or cured. Economic status no doubt plays a significant role in life expectancy. Certainly those with the resources to afford proper medical care fare far better than those who do not. Given each of us has a different economic status the overly simplistic answer to solve this dilemma would be to avoid illness and disease in the first place. We know there are no certainties in life nor are we born with a written guarantee. There are steps all of us can take, however, to significantly increase our chances for a longer, healthier life and to reduce the risk of disease. This leads us to the first and most important foundational concept to improve your odds for living longer and in better health:

Leading a sedentary lifestyle is a recipe for premature aging. If you believe proper exercise and nutrition will not make a difference by improving the chance to live longer and in better health you have been totally and completely misinformed.

This statement should be obvious, but it never ceases to amaze me how many people do not consider these critical factors in their day-to-day life. As a child I remember how insistent my parents were that I brush my teeth and get regular dental checkups. My parents lost their teeth at an early age due to the lack of dental care and were determined their children would not meet the same fate. It worked. I presume most people brush their teeth on a daily basis. Our teeth, however, represent only a fraction of our total body mass. Do you think the rest of our body does not need the same diligent care? What about our bones, joints, muscles, heart, lungs, and other organs? Do you think as we age they will care for themselves? Again, if you believe your body can sustain itself automatically and can run on any fuel you put in it, you have been totally and completely misinformed.

Certainly there are exceptions. Someone will always tell me they know 90-year-old Joe who smokes, drinks, eats pizza every day and is in perfect health. It's true; there are people on the planet who can live a long and perfectly healthy life being sedentary and on a poor diet, just as there are those who can live healthy lifestyles, exercise regularly and succumb at an early age. These are the extremes on the bell curve of life. Yet these percentages are so minute that for the vast majority of us such exceptions will not apply. A sedentary lifestyle and poor diet are like playing a football game in the middle of a busy freeway. As Dirty Harry actor, Clint Eastwood, once asked "are you feelin' lucky?" Smoking, drug and alcohol abuse, and obesity will also put you smack in the middle of the same freeway. You'll need a lot of luck to avoid the big semi that will almost certainly run right over you.

Finding who might be to blame for this epidemic of poor fitness and obesity in our society is senseless. Shakespeare probably explained it the best. "The fault, dear Brutus, is not in our stars, but in ourselves......." If there was one event that contributed to this trend, however, my vote would be the invention of the refrigerator. Why? Before the early 20th century (only a short time ago on the clock of human biological history) most people did not have a place to store food for long periods of time (though some city dwellers had "ice boxes" which had to be refilled every few days with large blocks of ice). Before that, salt was used to preserve most foods. People had to expend energy (calories) for every meal by hunting or gathering. Once the "fridge" came along it became all too easy to eat without expending energy. While certainly there are many other factors involved, is it any wonder so many people have gained weight when they spend virtually no energy to get their food?

A sedentary life and associated weight gain combine to create the perfect storm for disease and premature aging. Heart disease and several forms of cancer have been linked to these poor lifestyle choices.

Getting older does not mean an automatic ticket to the old age home! We can significantly increase our chance for an active, vibrant and healthy life well into our 80s and even 90s with the proper nutrition and exercise regimen.

If you think age is your limitation, guess again. We need only look at the feat accomplished by 64-year-old Diana Nyad in September, 2013, swimming over 100 miles from Cuba to Key West, Florida. I'm sure her genetics played a great part in this feat, but so did nutrition and proper training that expanded her physical boundaries to enable her to accomplish a life long goal. The only limitations we have are those we artificially create with the perception of our physical capabilities.

The fact is, training and nutrition are at the core of living a longer, healthier and more vibrant life. You may, however, be wondering if you have to train as hard as Diana Nyad to do so. Not exactly, but you can't sit in your easy chair either. We'll explore how much effort it takes in Chapter 7.

I believe most people wish for a disease free and pain free life with enough strength and vitality to do all the things they desire. Sounds great, yes! Unfortunately, this description is missing a very critical factor. It has to be sustainable! If you can't maintain your health over the years (and I mean decade after decade), is it really good health? If you took your car in for repair and your mechanic said "your car is fixed, but I'm not sure it will last another month or two," would you be a satisfied customer? Your health is no different.

CHAPTER 2

FIVE FACTORS THAT INFLUENCE YOUR HEALTH & LONGEVITY

Living a healthy, vibrant life requires recognizing many biological and physiological factors that affect our ability to resist disease and bodily decay. Only five factors, however, are relevant to our day-to-day living. Understand and manage these factors and your odds for living longer and healthier should improve significantly:

1. Your genetics
2. External factors
3. The food you eat
4. The quantity and quality of specific exercises
5. Mindfulness

Factor #1 is your heredity, your DNA. At the moment there is not much you can do about the genes you've inherited although modern science is making remarkable progress. Today it is relatively common to have heart, liver, and kidney transplants, and perhaps in time we'll even be able to regenerate organs and other body parts. Stem cell research is doing some amazing things so there is hope. However, the availability of genetic information is changing the way we behave and the options available to us. For now, what you can do is to know as much about your genetic history as you can, especially if you are predisposed to certain type of cancers, heart disease or other serious conditions. Risks cannot be eliminated, but they can certainly be reduced. Just ask Angelina Jolie who endured a double mastectomy and then had her ovaries and fallopian tubes removed after learning her genetics were almost certain to result in cancer.

Factor #2 is all things external. This includes blunt force trauma, exposure to carcinogens, radiation, auto accidents, falls, lightning strikes, earthquakes, avalanche, tsunamis, tornados, stray bullets, falling space debris, sink holes and other varieties of bad luck. Many of these events are not under your control, but others are clearly avoidable. One obvious example is drinking and driving. Another, but not so obvious example is this: In 2010, according to the Centers for Disease Control, 21,700 older adults died from falls.[3] Every hour of every day someone in the United States dies from homicide and another dies from a fall—both are American tragedies. By improving lower body strength, balance and some sensory re-education (see Chapter 8, For Seniors) there's a good chance the risk of falls can be reduced!

Factor #3 is the food you eat, and it's huge. You should have the proper amount and ratio of macro (carbohydrates, proteins and fats) and micro (vitamins and minerals) nutrients for proper cellular function. Chapters 5 & 6 describe the nutritional conditions that can help manage your weight and body fat.

Factor #4 is proper exercise. Surprise!! Let's be clear about this. My definition of exercise is not a walk each day in the park, although I'd be the last one to tell you not to walk. Someone told me recently that if walking was really that good for you every Postal Service Mail Carrier would be immortal. Don't misinterpret my views on walking, it's just that regular walking is like changing the oil in your car. If you don't change the oil, you may compromise the internal parts of your engine, so don't stop walking. Your transmission, brakes, tires, filters, etc., however, require periodic maintenance. So walking is "a good thing" as Martha Stewart might say, but it is only one of several things you need to do to maintain your health and extend your life. Remember, walking is not a cardiovascular improvement event unless you can sustain your heart rate (the number of beats per minute) in the range of 55 percent to 85 percent of its maximum (calculated by subtracting your age from 220).[4]

Example: You are 60 years old. Your maximum heart rate would be 220 minus 60 or 160. Therefore, sustaining a heart rate between 88-136 beats per minute for 20-40 minutes about three times per week should improve your cardiovascular fitness and help burn body fat if practiced on a continuing basis. If your heart rate falls below this range during exercise, you will certainly burn some calories but your cardiovascular system will not be getting enough stress for adaptive improvement. If your heart rate exceeds 85 percent of its maximum on a sustained basis other metabolic events can occur (i.e., to provide energy at this level your body will begin to burn additional protein as fuel). This means your metabolism will begin to disassemble your muscle and organ tissue for its energy needs which over time will lead to reduced muscle mass and loss of strength.

Yet, many marathon runners do this on a regular basis. Is it therefore unhealthy? The short answer is this: if practiced on a long term basis it's very good for your cardiovascular system, but not so good for your bones, joints and muscles. It's a trade off. We'll talk a bit more about this in Chapter 8 (For Runners).

> If you believe walking is the only exercise you need to do to stay healthy, fit and extend your life you have been misinformed. You should devote three to five hours per week to both anaerobic and aerobic exercise (about two percent to three percent of your total week), to positively affect your health, fitness and longevity.

Training with aerobic activities, which keep our heart rate at a sustained level, and anaerobic exercises, which include resistance and weight training, is a great way to improve health and wellness. It's not a guarantee of course. Risks will remain, but by consistently doing these activities your body's metabolism will adapt and you'll have more energy, be able to manage your weight, and have more strength and flexibility. Chapter 7 illustrates a sample program that can be used to make both strength and metabolic gains.

Your brain and your body are not separate. You may have noticed your neck connects the two and whatever happens below is going to have some impact on what happens above, and vice versa. Positive thought patterns and a balanced emotional life are important factors in sustaining health. Please refer to the section in Chapter 8 (The Magic of Mindfulness) for ideas about how to use your brain to positively affect your long term health and wellness.

Another important distinction is the difference between Health and Fitness. It is possible you can be healthy i.e., you are disease and pain free, but lack endurance, strength and flexibility. On the other side of the coin, you can have strength, endurance and flexibility, but have some type of disease (cancer, for example). While fitness always has a positive impact on your health, it is not a guarantee, just as good health does not guarantee your fitness.

> The pathway to good health is always a sound fitness and nutritional program.

In a nutshell, an effective fitness and nutritional lifestyle should achieve the following:

1. Cardio-respiratory efficiency;
2. Proper metabolic management: the ability to use carbohydrates, proteins and fats efficiently including the management of blood pressure, cholesterol level, blood sugar level and other critical metabolic and hormonal functions;
3. Maintaining or improving lean muscle mass for improved energy storage and endurance;
4. Maintaining or improving structural and postural integrity by properly exercising bones and joints (and thereby reducing the risk of injury);
5. Managing "sarcopenia" (age related loss of muscle mass) through strength training which has been shown to reduce the risk of osteopo-

rosis, arthritis, diabetes, and certain forms of cancer as well as improving energy and stamina;

6. Maintaining or improving flexibility (the range of motion around our joints);

7. A healthy immune system.[5]

Eating sensibly (i.e., a diet low in saturated fat with adequate protein, high in fiber and low in refined sugars and sodium) is always a good start, but by adding a regular program of strength training and cardiovascular exercise you can significantly alter your biological aging clock. *This is not a guess, nor a myth, nor marketing hype. It's the truth.*

Not convinced? Not a believer? Is it because you know an old Joe who's never worked out a day in his life and is a healthy 90-year-old? Or is it because it's too much effort? Or maybe because you think you don't have the time? Or perhaps, like so many people I encounter—you seem to be healthy enough even without exercise and a proper diet.

A scene in the movie "Batman Returns" features the Penguin (a hideous character played by actor Danny DeVito) who comes out of the sewer of Gotham

If you believe your health is sustainable without a proper diet and the right kind of exercise, you will find the above seven factors of good health very difficult to achieve. The result will be increasing your chances of acquiring age-related disease or disability and decreasing your chances of living a longer, healthier life.

City. The first person he meets is the Police Chief to whom the Penguin informs, "I'm going be the new Mayor." Of course the Police Chief tells him that's preposterous, but the Penguin replies, "things change!" Managing change is the major factor in how we should approach our health and well being.

If right now you feel great, it would be a huge mistake to think this is a permanent condition. Look down at your finger nail. You can't see it growing, can you? Certainly you know it grows because in a few days it will need to be clipped. Other changes in our bodies take quite a bit longer. Many cancers form slowly. Arthritis often takes years to show its effect, the same goes for heart disease.

In a nut shell, it is likely you will deteriorate just like a car that has not been properly maintained. Can't picture yourself as sick, old or frail? Just like a fingernail, you're going to get clipped unless you have a plan to manage the changes which are already taking place. Once again, this is not conjecture, a marketing ploy or a wild guess. You are going to change with age and that's the reality, but the process can be managed.

CHAPTER 3

ARE YOU AS TOUGH AS CHUCK?

Perhaps you are familiar with the legendary martial arts expert and actor, Chuck Norris. A few years ago someone started compiling a list of Chuck Norris facts designed to describe his "tough guy" persona. For example, why does Chuck Norris sleep with the light on? Answer: because the darkness is afraid of him. My most favorite is why doesn't Chuck Norris wear a watch? Answer: Chuck decides what time it is!

In terms of your health, this remark is what the British might say is "spot on." Each of us must decide what time it is in our life in terms of our health and wellness. By now you get the idea that a good diet and a sound, personalized exercise program are at the top of my list. Yes, it takes effort. Yes, it takes discipline. Yes, it takes time and toil. You have the option of taking control of your health or you can let your health take control of you. It's no different than having a hole in the bottom of your boat. If you don't bail water you will sink.

A personal observation: I have had friends and relatives over the years who acquired Alzheimer's disease. It's not a pleasant way to spend the golden years of your life. What is most interesting to me is every one of these people I knew lived sedentary lives. So far, I know of no one who has consistently trained with a combined aerobic and anaerobic program to suffer from Alzheimer's. Not having perfect knowledge, it is likely there are some. I did hear of a woman who was a long term runner who contracted this disease. I am hopeful more research will be conducted into the prevention of Alzheimer's through proper diet with the combined practice of both aerobic and anaerobic fitness. While the latest information from the medical community clearly indicates a regular fitness program has a positive effect on this terrible disease, only time will tell when or if a specific exercise and diet regimen can be developed that might target its prevention. In the mean time, my own personal experience says proper nutrition combined with regular aerobic and anaerobic exercise is a wise approach.

Of course, it is one thing to decide to do something and it is another to actually do it. Many people make the decision to get fit but somehow, someway it doesn't actually happen. Still others have almost every type of excuse known to man such as:

1. I don't have the time.
2. It's too much effort
3. I'm too tired
4. I can't afford a gym membership
5. I'm too old
6. what does it matter, I'm going to die of something anyway

What it boils down to is this: How much risk are you willing to take with the quality and length of your own life? The key factor that holds many people back from pursuing regular exercise and a proper diet as a course of action is they do not perceive an imminent threat to their well-being. The mistake is not recognizing the progression process of aging. The fatal flaw is thinking the past is a good predictor of the future—everything is ok now so it will be ok tomorrow too. There is no panic button to press until you contract a disease that may threaten your life or you realize you can't even walk up a flight of stairs without huffing and puffing.

I often get clients who come to me in their 60s, 70s or even 80s with frail, worn out bodies and want a fitness regimen that will take away their aches and pains. While it's never too late to make improvements, reversing many age-related conditions is not possible. The message here is obvious: do not put off a regular wellness program.

I knew a man who smoked all his life and had a series of heart attacks beginning at age 50. In his early 60s he had a massive heart attack, and a by-pass operation saved his life. He didn't quit smoking because he knew we all will die of something, besides he really enjoyed the smoking habit. In his early 70s he had a stroke and lost most of his eyesight. He lived in poor health until he was 78 when he died of lung cancer. The last 15 years of his life were basically spent as an invalid; he did not get to experience an active, healthy and vibrant retirement. This person was my father. He is not an exception. There are hundreds of thousands if not millions just like him who didn't make the most of the gift we could be blessed with—a healthy, vibrant and energetic life.

CHAPTER 4

SO, WHERE DO I BEGIN?

Just to refresh your memory, the pathway to a fitness and health improvement plan at any age always begins with your medical provider. *You must ensure you are healthy enough and have medical clearance to begin an exercise program in order to understand the contraindications, if any, of your particular situation*. Remember, any negative underlying conditions can trigger a dangerous if not fatal series of events. Getting a complete physical exam and blood workup is always the best course of action before beginning a training regimen.

When I train anyone I make it a practice to take my clients' blood pressure first. I've had several individuals with blood pressure so high I suggested they see their physician immediately. I wish this would be standard practice in the many gyms and fitness centers around the country. While heart attacks and strokes are rare at fitness centers, I know of several cases where fatalities have occurred while training that possibly could have been avoided if the victims and their trainers had understood the severity of their hypertension before engaging in a strenuous workout.

A shortcut is a method or procedure used to reduce time or energy expended. It is an American heritage. Some say this term has British origins. The term "rat running" or "cut-through" driving was used in the old days to describe people who cut through residential areas to avoid congested main roads. Regardless of origin, it has become almost an American cultural value to find shortcuts to save time and energy.

Unfortunately, shortcuts have found their way into the world of fitness. From 10-minute training sessions to wrapping our waists with elastic bands to promote weight loss, the marketers of the world are trying to convince us there are easier, faster and less energy-intensive ways to get fit. To figure out where to take the shortcuts, however, science rules the day. As previously mentioned, training your cardiovascular system to function properly and use oxygen efficiently, takes approximately 30 minutes of exercise at a level of 55 percent to 85 percent of your maximum heart rate (MHR) about three times per week. That's about as much of a shortcut as you are going to get if you want your cardiovascular system to work most efficiently.[6]

I am often asked about 10-minute training regimens. Are they effective? My short answer is they are certainly better than being sedentary, but I think you'll find even these programs will encourage you to do more than the basic 10 minutes. When you do the minimum of anything you will get minimal results. Make sure you read the fine print first before you buy any packaged fitness routine or equipment. Remember, most of the marketing is to get you to buy the product. I will note one exception for those who are already in top physical shape. The Tabata protocols, i.e., 4- minute high- intensity training segments, 20 seconds at

100 percent effort followed by 10 seconds of rest for eight intervals, has been shown to be a highly effective conditioning routine which takes only four minutes. Please understand this should only be attempted by those who are very physically fit since it demands pushing your cardiovascular system to very high limits, but as shortcuts go, this training sequence appears to be the real deal.

If you have not trained before, I suggest you first get your cardiovascular system in shape by beginning slowly. Start by walking at a pace that is most comfortable but as fast as you can reasonably go. If you can do five minutes then do five minutes. Work yourself up to 30 minutes at least three times per week. Remember, the secret is getting your heart rate to a sustained level (i.e., between 55 percent and 85 percent of your maximum heart rate). Once you are at this level, then progress to adding strength training to your routine. Strength training is discussed in Chapter 7. Before we get you pumping iron, however, let's review nutritional needs and the basics of weight management.

CHAPTER 5

DIET & NUTRITION: CONTROL YOUR WEIGHT/CONTROL YOUR LIFE

Thousands of books have been written about diet and nutrition. In some way, shape or form diet is always in the news, internet, magazines, billboards, and the Food Channel on a daily basis. Rather than give you a plethora of diet methodologies and recipes, I am giving you the short course on weight management so you don't have to sift through mountains of conflicting studies and claims in the media.

Many regularly marketed diet and nutrition programs will get you to lose weight initially, but few have a process that allows you to maintain your loss. Once you're off the plan you can easily bounce back into the no man's land of weight gain. Some programs want you to keep paying for them long after you've lost weight. A recent Consumer Reports study revealed that of the major diet plans on the market the "Best of the Best" had only a 19 percent success rate (defined as those who reached their targeted weight loss goal). [7] Let's explore some concepts that could make a difference for you.

The basics of nutrition are actually quite simple. Our body needs substrates, i.e., macronutrients (carbohydrates, proteins and fats) to supply energy. Carbohydrates are the essential fuel in the form of glucose that run our muscles and provide the required energy for our brain and central nervous system. Proteins, which are made of amino acids, are used primarily for hormone and enzyme development and organ, tissue and structural repair (bones, cartilage, etc). Fats are used to transport certain fat-soluble vitamins (A, D, E & K), balance hormones, form cellular membranes and store energy. Each of these macronutrients has a vital function for your metabolism. Micronutrients (vitamins and minerals) on the other hand, have zero energy value but are fundamental to energy transfer and cellular function and must be present in sufficient quantities to do their job. [8]

The traditional weight management concept and the first law of thermodynamics state that if you take in more calories than your body uses you will gain weight. Take in fewer calories than your body uses and you will lose weight. One pound of body fat is equivalent to about 3500 calories. So in one week, let's say you take in 3500 calories more than you burn, you would put on approximately one pound. One would like to believe that's the end of the story but it's not that simple. Other forces are at play that affect the outcome of your weight gain or loss.

While the math is simple, the human body is not. The components of our genetics make weight loss and gain much more complex and difficult to manage. Some people have a naturally high metabolism and do not gain weight easily.

Others have a very slow metabolism and gain weight on the same caloric intake as the person with the higher metabolism. Then there are diets, like Atkins, that recommend restricting carbohydrates to get you to lose weight faster. Atkins contends that by restricting carbohydrate intake your body will use the next available fuel source—fat. While the low carb strategy has logic, the number of calories you burn is still a factor. If you take on too many calories in the form of protein or fat, your body may still store the excess calories, depending on how your individual metabolism works. Another critical factor is the type of carbohydrates Atkins recommends removing from your diet. Carbs with high sugar content i.e., those with a high glycemic index, make a significant difference in weight loss or gain.[9]

Science Writer Gary Taubes explains the majority of weight loss will come from the reduced intake of refined carbohydrates due to their effect on insulin levels.[10] There is also another factor, at least in initial phases of weight loss that comes into play—water. With each gram of glycogen bound to three or four grams of water, a very low carbohydrate diet, which effectively depletes your stores of glycogen, will cause water to be used in this depletion, and hence, initial weight loss can occur somewhat faster. If you go back to having a positive energy balance, i.e., you store more calories than you burn, weight gain from water will return. The key factor appears to be hormonal. Excess sugar in the diet causes insulin to be released and this hormone seems to be a major factor in controlling the amount of fat that is stored or burned. So, even though you might take in fewer calories you may not burn them as fast resulting in weight gain. From my personal experience

Atkins and Taubes have it right which is why I am a huge fan of low refined sugar diets.

Sedentary individuals can benefit from low carbohydrate diets because they don't use as many carbs as active people. So if you are "activity restricted" for whatever reason, a low carb diet is an excellent way of managing weight gain, however, overload on proteins and fats and you might not see positive results. Active people need a certain level of carbohydrates for their bodies to function properly, but indeed Atkins and Taubes offer a powerful message: too many "empty carbs", i.e., sugars that are quickly digested and play havoc with your insulin levels, are to be avoided. Eating fresh vegetables, with fiber-based carbs that are absorbed more slowly, is different from eating candy bars that cause a more rapid rise in blood glucose levels.

Since all of us have different metabolic rates, I am a firm believer in the "trial and error" approach when it comes to how many carbohydrates, proteins and fats you should consume. If you are highly active (either through workouts, sports, or your particular job or profession) then a diet consisting of 50 percent carbohydrates, 33 percent proteins and 17 percent fats may be a good fit. If you are less active then 40 percent carbohydrates, 40 percent protein and 20 percent fats is likely better. Adjustments to these "rule of thumb" percentages can only be made based on how you feel and the results you get after applying them. If you have a regular workout program or engage in an energy intensive sport you will need more carbohydrates depending on how much energy your muscles use. If you are less active, your body will not use as many carbohydrates so you might consider beginning at the 40% carb level and adjusting up or down depending on how you feel and what your weight and body fat goals might be. Very low carb, low calorie or liquid diets should be monitored by your health care provider or a certified nutritionist. These dietary options may be appropriate for the morbidly obese, but can be dangerous if not closely managed.

Even if you are the type who does not like counting calories or has no desire to track your carbohydrate, protein and fat percentages, don't worry. Chapter 6 describes the DGOLF Diet plan which can be used to trim pounds by making a few strategic adjustments. You'll be able to shed pounds slowly but regularly by cycling your calories, lowering your sodium intake and managing the amount of "empty" carbohydrate calories you consume, i.e. refined sugars.

The DGOLF plan is designed to help you lose weight, but it is also a way of managing your nutrition for the long term. Diets in themselves are most often restrictive and many feel deprived of their favorite foods which can result in "diet depression." This can also explain why people who come off their diets tend to regain much if not all of the weight they lost. The DGOLF plan does restrict you for four consecutive days but allows your favorites to come back on the fifth day.

My principles behind weight management are scientific and not new. Many of the proven and practical weight loss methods seem to get lost somewhere between the information overload we are subjected to each day, and slick and often misleading weight-loss product advertising. For those interested in detailed scientific nutritional information I suggest reading the works of sports nutritionist Dr. Dan Benardot, science writer Gary Taubes, and medical doctor and a founder of the Nutrition Science Initiative, Dr. Peter

Attia, who have contributed significantly to nutritional science and weight management.

Let's review some basic weight loss concepts: The traditional metabolic rule of thumb says it takes about 3500 calories to lose one pound. Without counting all the calories we eat each day, let's start by just reducing our daily caloric intake by 300 calories (skip the daily bagel or another carbohydrate-based food that equals 300 calories). Then, try to burn another 300 calories by some form of caloric burn (a 30 minute bike ride for example). Therefore, in seven days you should use about 4200 calories and lose a bit more than a pound. If you didn't, you can change the equation by adding another reduction in caloric intake and by increasing the amount of exercise until you do lose the pound. This trial and error process is a practical way to determine what works for you. The math says you could achieve the same results by restricting your daily caloric intake by 600 and not exercising at all (not a recommended option), or keep your caloric intake the same and increase your calorie burn by 600 calories (not a bad option).

Please note this process will work only until your body discovers it is on a pathway to starvation (i.e., your body will not let you lose weight indefinitely). If you want to continue to lose weight your metabolism must be reset to avoid metabolic slowdown. To do this you should "cycle" your calories periodically. The method I find most effective is restricting caloric intake for four consecutive days. Then on the fifth day come off this restriction—go ahead and eat your bagel. This should convince your metabolism that you are not on a diet and you can outsmart what is normally called the "plateau effect."

The next chapter has more about the DGOLF diet including a "Foods to Avoid" list. These every day foods are either high in sugar, salt, saturated fat or calories and will sabotage your weight loss goals. Avoid them! The basic DGOLF diet is quite easy to follow. There are just these simple behaviors: Cycle calories every fifth day, don't eat what's on the "Foods to Avoid" list and do the recommended workout outlined in Chapter 7.

Many people are refined sugar addicts (chocolate, ice cream, cakes, pies, donuts, etc.) and have a very difficult time eliminating the products on the "Foods to Avoid" list. A number of options can help. Several brands of snack products have replaced sugar with sugar alcohols. Sorbitol and Maltitol are commonly used to replace sugar, have about half the calories of sugar and do not contribute to tooth decay. While these sugar replacements have been deemed safe, taken in excess they can potentially cause gastric distress (gas and bloating are the most common). Used in moderation, they can be a replacement for the sweet tooth, but may have some side effects.

Many fans of the recently popular "Paleo Diet" might frown upon using sugar substitutes because they are not "natural" per se, but eliminating significant sugar intake from the diet is the prime directive. Certainly in a perfect world it would be better not to consume sugar alcohols, but it's likely a good interim step in transitioning to a more natural diet. While I like the concept of the natural foods, the Paleo plan™ excludes whole grains and dairy which have considerable nutrient value and are excellent sources of Vitamin C and D.

Ok, so would it be possible to lose weight by eating just 1000 calories a day of pizza and ice cream? The math may say so, but your health is not sustainable without all the proper macro and micronutrients. You might lose weight, but with a diet high in fat and carbohydrates and lacking many vitamins and minerals you would soon suffer a variety of symptoms associated with vitamin and mineral deficiency including fatigue, nausea, gastrointestinal distress, dermatitis, dementia, diarrhea, sleeplessness, depression, anemia, neurological problems, impaired blood clotting and more.

The best way to avoid nutritional deficiency and manage your weight, is to just eat foods that are nutrient dense and include a wide variety of fruits, vegetables, seeds and nuts, lean protein, low fat dairy and whole grains. You can also limit the amount of sugary carbohydrates, particularly if you are sedentary. If you are physically very active, understand our bodies require a significant amount of carbohydrates for brain and muscle function, plus at higher activity levels, if you don't get enough carbs, you will be burning fat as the next available fuel. The process to convert fat into glycogen for energy is a bit more involved than using muscle glycogen so it is possible you may feel a bit sluggish and less energetic at first. Again, only trial and error will determine the minimum amount of carbohydrates necessary to operate your particular metabolism, but as a general rule the more physically active you are the more carbohydrates you will need.

I also strongly advise against losing weight without a strength training program. Why? Because while you may be losing

> Weight loss without resistance training to replace lost muscle mass will only serve to make you weaker in the long run.

weight, you're not just losing all fat—you're losing muscle fiber as well.

Strength training should be fundamental to any diet. Unfortunately most diet plans completely avoid this important step. You *must* do strength training if you want to avoid sarcopenia (age-related loss of muscle mass). *This is not a guess. This is not a myth. This is not marketing hype. This is scientific fact.*[11]

But exactly how many calories do *you* need each day? We are all of different size, shape and metabolic rate. There are several ways to calculate your caloric need. The more scientific methods (indirect and direct calorimetry) are not very practical since they must be performed in a laboratory. Several mathematical equations, however, can provide a reasonable estimate.

Knowing your RMR (the number of calories per day you consume while at rest) can give you an excellent starting place to managing body weight (refer to Chapter 6 for the Owen equation calculation). Be aware, however, individual genetic and metabolic differences can skew caloric equations.

People with higher body fat often have a lower RMR, and those with higher muscle content would likely have a higher RMR. Some people may have ultra slow or ultra fast metabolisms and the RMR calculation may not be accurate. The best way to understand your true caloric utilization is to monitor your caloric intake over time, weigh yourself regularly, and track your activity level. The combination of caloric intake and activity level will yield either a positive or negative energy balance and you'll gain weight, lose weight or stay the same.

If you have difficulty controlling your food intake, to lose weight you will need to increase your exercise regimen. If you are disciplined enough to limit your calories, you will lose weight faster by increasing your level of exercise. Weight management is a combination of art and science because you have multiple options of combining your food intake with caloric burning methods, i.e., aerobic and anaerobic exercise. If aerobics is your only method of exercise, you might lose weight if you burn more calories than you take in, but long term you will become weaker and less flexible because you will be losing muscle fiber to sarcopenia.

The world of sports is no longer a game, but a huge money-making business. Professional and amateur athletes alike strive for the best human performance possible. Training methods have become more and more scientific and sports science has advanced to heights previously thought to be science fiction. World records in many competitive sports continue to be broken as nutritional and training techniques improve. Proper muscular development, training for the maximum use of oxygen, and proper diets are not just for professional

> The proper way to manage your weight is through a combination of proper nutrition with both aerobic and anaerobic exercise. This will ensure you are caring for both your cardiovascular system (using aerobics) and your muscles, bones and joints (using anaerobics) as well as improving your body's overall metabolic capability. This is not a guess. This is not a myth. This is not marketing hype. This is scientific fact.

athletes—they're for all of us at every age and can make our lives more productive, healthier and more energetic.

CHAPTER 6

WEIGHT MANAGEMENT: THE DGOLF DIET

(It's not just for Golfers!)

In a nutshell, below are the basic principles of the DGOLF diet, a common sense plan for managing your weight at any age. Please note this diet is not meant to treat any specific disease or other medical condition. It is designed only for weight management and the benefits derived from attaining an appropriate weight. The five specific food categories, including the important "foods to avoid" list that follows, are the core of the DGOLF plan.

D	Dairy	the low fat kind (skip butter, cream, whole milk, and full fat cheeses).
G	Grains	whole grains with plenty of fiber (skip the whole wheat and multi-grain varieties which may have been robbed of their bran nutrients and fiber)

O	Oils	rich in mono and polyunsaturated fatty acids, antioxidants and vitamins (like Olive, Avocado, Coconut, Walnut, Peanut and Grapeseed oils)
L	Lean meats, chicken, turkey and fish	skip the processed meats and farm raised fish
F	Fruits and Vegetables, Nuts & Seeds	eat four servings of veggies for every one serving of fruit

The dynamics of weight gain and loss vary with each individual. Physiological considerations combined with careful planning are necessary to achieve desired results. For many, it is managing calories in and calories out, for others it has much to do with the hormone insulin and intake of carbohydrates, especially refined sugars. Exercise also plays a significant role. Each of us has a different metabolic rate, different genetics and hormonal sensitivity. Therefore, it is critical to consider these factors:

1. The total number of calories you consume (in the form of carbohydrates, proteins and fats);
2. Your individual metabolic rate (combination of genetics and lifestyle);
3. The quantity and quality of exercise you engage in (which affects metabolic rate);
4. The sensitivity to insulin and other metabolic hormones in your system;
5. The thermic effect of food* and the uptake of nutrients to the blood.

* The thermic effect of food refers to the calories burned in the diges-tion process, normally about 10 percent of total caloric intake. Sugars require little digestion and hence, by eating too many sugars, much of the thermic effect is lost.

WEIGHT MANAGEMENT

Start a log book and weigh yourself every two to three days. If you are under 21 it is possible you are still in a growth mode so weight and muscle gain are to be expected. If you calculate your Body Mass Index (BMI) as shown on page 56, it will give you a general idea of where you are on the obesity scale.

Please note BMI is only a broad screening calculation. Individuals with large frames may not score well using this method. BMI must be combined with other factors includ-ing body fat percentage, lean muscle mass and blood and hormonal indicators to more properly understand ideal weight and body composition. From a fitness perspective, higher body fat percentages have been linked to increased risk of heart disease, certain types of cancers, diabetes and other illnesses.

If you are a young athlete, ideal body fat percentages can vary depending on the sport you play. Unless you are an elite athlete (an Olympian perhaps) body fat under 8 percent is questionable. While body fat percentage is only one aspect indicating the efficiency of your metabolic system, it is high on my list of controllable factors.

For males 18 and older a good rule of thumb is a body fat range of 8 to19 percent and for females 21 to 32 percent. Since body frames and height vary, these ranges are only general guidelines, and being height/weight appropriate is often a matter of personal preference. Body fat tends to increase as we age, so a 65-year-old would not be expected to have the same body fat percentage as a 25-year- old (add about one percent per decade).

As an example, a 45–year-old male might range between 11 and 21 percent and a 65-year- old between 13 and 24 percent.[12] Given the many health factors involved, however, it is always wise to review your weight and body fat goals with your physician.

So how are body fat measurements taken? Most certified fitness trainers use either calipers or instruments that employ bioelectrical impedance to calculate body fat and lean muscle mass. While they are not as accurate as clinical methods, they can give you a reasonable indication of your body composition. You can also consult your physician who can arrange a calculation. Body weight/body fat scales using bioelectrical impedance can be purchased at department stores.

FOR WEIGHT LOSS

To lose weight, the DGOLF diet guidelines are listed below, but it always takes discipline to succeed in reaching any goal. If you follow these steps in about a week you should be able to adapt to the physical and psychological changes and begin losing weight. If this does not happen you will need to make further adjustments to the diet and/or exercise plan.

It is important to review any dietary or exercise changes with your health care provider before adopting a weight loss (or gain) program. While it is unlikely your physician would object to improvements in your nutrition, exercise intensity or frequency, your individual circumstance may be such that some or all of the DGOLF diet plan and associated exercises may not be appropriate for you.

THE DGOLF DIET GUIDELINES

1. Pick an item(s) of approximately 300 calories you normally eat and eliminate it from your diet for four consecutive days. For example, if you have a bagel and cream cheese each day, drop it from your diet.

2. Every fifth day add this item or an equivalent 300 calories back in your diet. It is important on day five you take in about 15 percent more calories than you took in on days one through four. Your body must periodically reset itself otherwise it will think you are dieting and your metabolism will slow down. Then start over with the reduced caloric intake while closely following the "foods to avoid" list. Do this for another four consecutive days and so on. Use this process until you reach your desired weight/body fat percentage.

3. Control your intake of simple sugars. *Read food labels.* If it says more than five grams of sugar—avoid it. While there are no formal guidelines for sugar on nutrition labels, I suggest keeping intake to no more than 20-25 grams per day, even less is better. If you are diabetic, check with your physician. If you do have an uncontrollable sweet tooth, as previously mentioned, there are sugar substitutes on the market that will not spike your insulin levels e.g., sugar alcohols. Please note some individuals may experience gastric distress with these sugar substitutes. Sugar intake will raise insulin levels and studies show this has an effect on the storage of fat

in our metabolism, so limiting sugar intake is critical to weight and metabolic management. *Avoid the following as they are either high in sodium, sugar, saturated fat or lack sufficient fiber:*

THE DGOLF FOODS TO AVOID LIST:

- fruit juices
- french fries
- white bread (choose "Whole Grain" products instead)
- whole milk products including butter and full fat cheeses (non-fat milk products OK)
- cakes
- pies
- pastries
- bagels
- pizza
- cream sauces
- cooking oils (olive, canola, grapeseed, walnut, coconut oils are OK)
- mayonnaise (low sugar mayo substitutes OK)
- fried foods
- chips
- canned vegetables
- sausage & hot dogs
- bacon, bologna, salami and processed meats
- creamy salad dressings
- pancakes and syrup
- pasta (high fiber pastas OK)
- soda (diet soda OK in very limited quantities)
- corn starch
- tortillas (high fiber varieties OK)

- white potatoes (sweet potatoes OK)
- white rice
- chocolate (sugar free chocolates OK)
- ice cream (low sugar yogurt or Greek Yogurt OK)
- most cereals (regular Cherrios® and shredded wheat OK or those with less than five grams of sugar)
- corn & peas (have in limited quantity as they have high sugar content)
- limit alcohol consumption to no more than three drinks per week

4. Fresh fruits and veggies are critical (try to keep them in a four to one ratio—eat four veggies to one fruit). Lean meats, turkey, chicken and fish are all good. Salads and soups are OK—just avoid canned soups with high sodium content, cream based soups and high calorie salad dressings. Whole grain bread is OK in limited quantity, but avoid whole wheat bread and multi-grain breads which may have been robbed of their nutrients by manufacturers who often extract the vital nutrients in the bran. Pasta is OK if it's whole grain, but no more than once or twice per week.

5. Do both aerobic and anaerobic workouts: three to five hours per week of training will get you the best results. See Chapter 7 for my suggested workout plan, and note the strategy is to practice strength training and aerobics on a regular basis (preferably at least three days per week). There is an excellent website (EXRX.net) that can provide guidance on how to begin a proper strength training program or find a competent personal trainer

who can show you the protocols and safety practices necessary to achieve the best results.

If you are not losing weight after the first week, do the following: 1) First, reduce your caloric intake by another 300 calories per day. 2) If you are still not losing weight after another week, add a 45-minute to one hour strength training workout to your weekly routine. 3) If still no weight loss, reduce caloric intake by another 200 calories per day. 4) If still no weight loss, increase the intensity of your workouts (increase weight and/or reps).

Please consider weight training will increase your muscle mass and while muscle and fat weigh the same (a pound is a pound), muscle has more density. Muscle also consumes calories on a sustained basis so you will be increasing your metabolic rate by adding muscle. You may initially gain a bit of weight through strength training but these gains should be minimal. You will be losing inches from key areas as your body changes and your metabolism improves.

THE VOICE OF REASON

Let's be real. It is unreasonable to expect you will be perfect in following the above plan. You don't have to. That's one of the advantages of Day Five. It's OK to have a couple of slices of pizza, ice cream or chocolate on the fifth day—just be disciplined for four out of five days and keep your portion sizes reasonable. Because the DGOLF diet is based on foods not to eat, this leaves a pretty wide open field of foods that are available to you. This does not mean, however, it is open season on everything. You cannot consume huge quantities of meat, fish, fruits or even healthy nutrient dense foods and expect to lose weight. You must use common sense and practice portion control. Don't eat until you feel stuffed.

Meat or fish in four to six oz. portions should be sufficient for almost everyone. By combining complex carbohydrates (as in most vegetables) with lean protein sources (as in lean chicken, turkey, fish, eggs or meat) at every meal, you will feel fuller and have fewer cravings. While fruit is an excellent source of vitamins and minerals and is high in fiber, it is also high in sugar content, which is why I recommend a ratio of four vegetables to one fruit. Please be aware the sugars in fruit are absorbed more slowly than sugars from fruit juice because of the higher fiber content, so following the four to one ratio will help manage your insulin levels to avoid metabolic slowdown. Remember it is critical to consume as few simple sugars as possible for four consecutive days of the program.

When embarking on the DGOLF diet some people may want more specific instructions and even planned menus. My diet is designed for flexibility and avoidance of poor food choices, but for those who want a bit more structure

> Strength training is critical to your success! Weight loss burns both fat and muscle tissue. Muscle must be replaced by strength training or you risk becoming weaker and more frail as you age. Sarcopenia (age related loss of muscle mass) is a serious condition that you want to avoid as you age, and until medical science finds an alternative, strength training is the only known answer!

please refer to the low calorie menu example later in this chapter. While it is only a one-day example of a bit over 1700 calories, it is illustrative of a very low carb diet. This would be a suggested plan for a female weighing about 120 pounds who has a fairly low activity level. This same person, however, with increased or decreased exercise levels could easily vary 300-500 calories in either direction. Activity levels, particularly strength training, require a higher amount of carbohydrates and calories to maintain weight. Some trial and error may be necessary to determine the exact number of calories that will fit your particular goal (i.e., to lose weight, gain weight or stay the same).

For those not wanting to count calories just follow the DGOLF diet plan as presented. It is also helpful to be prepared by shopping well ahead of time and making the best effort to eliminate the items on the "foods to avoid" list from your refrigerator and pantry.

Extra Fat-Loss option: Let's say you are going to workout at eight am. One option is to have breakfast after your workout. With fewer carbohydrates in your system this should cause you to burn additional fat. You can try this method for a bit faster fat loss, but see how your body reacts to having a shortage of carbohydrates which are in great demand during muscular exercise.

If you do eat, make sure to do so at least 30 minutes before working out. The digestive system shuts down when high demand is placed on muscular energy, and you may experience varying degrees of nausea if you eat too soon before a workout.

OTHER IMPORTANT TIPS:
- Eat something at least every three hours. Don't go hungry or you'll overeat.
- Eat protein <u>and</u> carbohydrates at every meal.
- Don't skip breakfast. Yogurt is not breakfast nor is a glass of orange juice (note: juices are on the "foods to avoid" list). Have an orange instead. It has the fiber that slows sugar absorption.
- Stay hydrated. Drink plenty of water especially during your workouts.
- Snacking during the day is essential. Don't go hungry. An apple, banana or some nuts is OK for between-meal snacks.
- Eat for activity. If you are going to expend energy you will need more calories than if you're just going to watch TV.
- Make the last meal of the day your lightest.
- Note the fiber content on the foods you are eating. Fiber is an important part of the digestive process and those under the age of 50 should aim for eating approximately 25 grams of dietary fiber each day for women and 38 grams for men. For the over-50 set the recommendations are 30 grams for men and 21 grams for women.[13]
- Brush your teeth and floss immediately after your dinner meal to discourage you from snacking in the evenings.

If you want to count calories and you plan to follow a regular workout program, start with a diet that is approximately 50 percent carbohydrates, 33 percent protein and 17 percent fat. The more strength training you do, the more carbohydrates your system will need. Trial and error may be necessary to determine the desired results.

How you feel is another important indicator of the proper combination of diet and exercise. Fatigue can be a result of diet deficiencies or over training, so closely monitor not only your weight but your energy levels as well. Fatigue can result in a compromised immune system and lead to colds, respiratory issues, etc. Rest is an important component of any exercise program, so make sure you take off some time from training each week (1-2 days), stay hydrated and get plenty of sleep.

If you have followed the plan and have reached your desired weight and body fat percentage, continue to weigh yourself regularly and adjust your diet accordingly. If you gain a couple of pounds, go back to the calorie cycling plan. If you have not been successful using the plan steps, it is possible your metabolic rate is very slow. You might need to be very specific on the number of calories you consume each day as well the amount of refined sugar intake. Look for these hidden sugars in your diet. Cut back a bit on fruits, which have natural sugars. Before making any drastic changes to your plan, however, consult your physician as certain medical conditions (like thyroid dysfunction) may be the root cause for failure to lose weight.

CALCULATING YOUR BODY MASS INDEX (BMI):

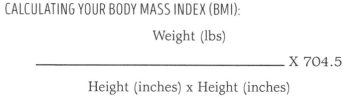

$$\frac{\text{Weight (lbs)}}{\text{Height (inches) x Height (inches)}} \text{ X } 704.5$$

<u>Example</u>: female 130 lbs 5 ft. 7 inches tall (67 inches) 130 divided by 67 X 67 = .02896 x 704.5 = **20.4 BMI**

NATIONAL INSTITUTE OF HEALTH-PERCENTAGE STANDARDS FOR BODY MASS INDEX

Normal	18.5-24.9%
Overweight	20.0-29.9%
Obesity class I	30.0-34.9%
Obesity Class II	35.0-39.9%
Extreme Obesity	≥ 40.0%

EXAMPLE LOW CARB, MODERATE CALORIE MENU

	Total Calories*	Protein	Carbs	Fat
BREAKFAST				
2 eggs scrambled	365	100	20	245
1 cup mixed fruit	60	3	55	2
8 oz. unsweetened Almond Milk	30	4	4	22
1 thin slice of whole grain bread	60	13	37	10
Coffee or tea (no sugar or cream)	0	0	0	0
SNACK				
Handful of Almonds	89	12	13	64
LUNCH				
1 cup water packed tuna fish	169	157	0	12
1 thin slice whole grain bread	60	13	37	10

	Total Calories*	Protein	Carbs	Fat
2 tbsp. mayo substitute	26	0	8	18
Small Caesar salad	200	20	36	144
SNACK				
1 cup carrot sticks, broccoli	49	8	36	5
3 oz. Hummus	144	27	93	24
DINNER				
5 oz. lean cut steak	239	104	0	135
1 cup grilled asparagus	32	12	20	0
Sliced tomato, medium	40	8	28	4
1 cup green beans, steamed	40	8	32	0
DESSERT				
1 cup low fat Greek yogurt	132	44	88	0
	1735	**533**	**507**	**695**
		30%	30%	40%

* Approximate values

Please note the above menu is for illustrative purposes only and is representative of a very low carb diet for weight loss. This would not be appropriate for everyone, especially athletes or those who engage in significant amounts of muscular exercise where carbohydrates are the main source of energy

If you wish to count calories using the DGOLF diet first calculate your RMR (resting metabolic rate), i.e., the number of calories you consume at rest for a 24-hour period. If you do nothing all day but watch TV, your body would use a certain number of calories just to maintain your body systems e.g., digestive, lymphatic, cardiovascular, etc. This will give you a base number to establish your minimum caloric needs. Once you know this number you can estimate the number of calories you require on a daily basis.

Remember, this is only an estimate and your actual RMR may be lower or higher depending on your individual metabolic rate.

The Owen Equation is one of the easier methods to calculate your RMR:

For men: RMR= 879+10.2 x weight in kilograms

For women RMR=795 +7.2 x weight in kilograms (a kilogram equals 2.204 pounds)

Example: a woman weighing 135 pounds (61 .3 kilograms) would have an RMR of 795+7.2 x 61.3 = 1236 calories per day.[14]

Therefore, a 135 lb. woman would burn 1236 calories at rest. If she had any muscular activity during the day (like walking, bike riding, weight lifting, etc.) and burned 400 calories doing these activities, her daily caloric need would be 1636 calories. If she ate more calories than this she would have a positive energy balance and would likely gain weight, or if she ate less than this amount she would have a negative energy balance and lose weight. If she ate exactly 1636 calories she would have a neutral energy balance and stay the same.

Using this method can help approximate your daily caloric intake to match your activity level and assist in designing a menu that should stimulate weight loss. Remember, this calculation is only an approximation and your individual metabolic rate will vary based on your actual diet, exercise regimen, hormones and other factors. Therefore, please check your weight and body fat percentage on a regular basis. If you are not losing weight please refer to the process described in #5 of the DGOLF diet guidelines.

CHAPTER 7

GET STRONGER, LIVE LONGER: THE WORKOUTS

The options are infinite when it comes to exercise. The human body is capable of both linear and non-linear motion and therefore movement has almost no bounds. If you've ever seen a performance of Cirque du Soleil you know what I mean. For workout enthusiasts, Men's Health® Magazine has published a book listing over 600 worthwhile exercises, but in fact, the list doesn't stop there.

The dilemma for most is choosing the right exercises and then finding the time to do them. The reality is we are in information overload which adds unnecessary complexity further complicated by marketers who are trying to take your money by convincing you their program is the best.

Then, there are just too many definitions and varieties of exercise. Some people become dedicated solely to stretching routines while others swear by yoga, Pilates, Zumba®, weight-lifting, CrossFit, running or tai chi—you name it. The real question is what effect do these different exercises have on your metabolism and body structure? For example, a regular stretching routine might make you a bit more nimble and improve or maintain your range of motion, but it will do almost nothing for your metabolism or your body's ability for oxygen uptake. Before you adopt a lifestyle using any one of these name brand exercises I encourage you to understand the full effect it can have on your body systems.

The objective is to achieve the seven lifestyle goals mentioned in Chapter 2, including metabolic fitness (your body's ability to use energy efficiently), structural integrity (full function of your muscles, bones and joints), and proper cardiovascular efficiency. If after diligent attention to this diet and exercise program you do not achieve these objectives then you likely need to reassess your fitness model, particularly if you want to lead a fully functional life in your golden years.

Any weakness in this chain and you will lose energy and mobility and open the door to increased risk of disease and frailty. I have seen too many people who thought they were doing the right thing by just being walkers, runners, or practicing yoga. If you want to achieve the best results, it is important not to be one-dimensional in your fitness routines.

My workout is designed to achieve functional performance by developing all your muscle groups. Followed correctly, these routines will make you stronger, improve core strength and enable you to adapt to whatever future level of fitness you may wish to pursue. Just remember to check with your physician before beginning any new workout routine. Strength training raises both blood pressure and heart rate and any underlying medical conditions can trigger a catastrophic series of events, so a medical exam before you begin is wise.

While the workout I propose is great for beginners, it can be used effectively at intermediate and advanced levels (with some adjustments discussed at the end of the chapter). It is designed specifically for muscular growth (hypertrophy) to improve overall strength and combat sarcopenia.

First, a few instructions and precautions:

1. Always warm up before you attempt to lift any weights. This means five to 10 minutes of walking on a treadmill, doing jumping jacks or other activities to induce a light sweat. Muscles need to get warm before being used strenuously. Active stretching is OK (swinging your arms or other fluid motions), but static stretching is not recommended during warm up. This means no pushing or pulling on your joints until you are fully warmed up.

2. Weight training is the most effective way to strengthen your muscles, bones and joints, but proper form is necessary to avoid injury. If you practice "segment alignment" you will significantly reduce the risk of injury and achieve maximum results. This means, for most every exercise, weight needs to be moved in a straight line away from your joint. Think of it this way, our bodies are designed in a straight line with our knees over our ankles, hips over our knees, shoulders over our hips. Weight training machines are designed to keep us in segment alignment. Moving free weights around (dumbbells, kettle bells and barbells), however, does not ensure segment alignment and must be done with caution. If you don't belong to a fitness center and/or don't have access to a certified fitness trainer, look for websites that can show you the proper form. The website EXRX.net is excellent. Go

to the Exercise and Muscle Directory to see short videos of exercises for each muscle group.

3. The proper training sequence is as follows:
    1. warm up (5-10 minutes)
    2. weight training exercises
    3. abdominal exercises
    4. stretching and cool down
    5. Cardiovascular (aerobic exercises which can be done on non-weight training days, if desired)

It is important to follow this sequence as weight training uses abdominal muscles for stabilization. Therefore, if you do abdominal work before your weight training your abs will be tired and you will be less effective. Similarly, if you do cardio before your weight training and burn some amount of carbohydrates, you will be less effective when doing weight training where carbohydrate needs are the highest.

4. The program recommended below includes three days per week of weight training e.g., Monday, Wednesday and Friday. It also includes cardio routines that cause you to elevate your heart rate for 20+ minutes at a time. Brisk walking, running or biking, for example, can be done after your weight training or on alternate non-weight training days. I suggest you take off at least one day per week to rest.

5. What's the proper weight for each exercise? This takes a bit of trial and error but you know you have the proper weight if you can complete each set when the last two or three repetitions are difficult, and you could only do two or

three more. If you get to the third set it's OK to reduce the weight as long as the last two or three repetitions are still difficult. On an effort scale of one to 10, where one is as easy as picking up a pencil and 10 is lifting something you can barely do, your effort level should be about an eight. This level of effort is the approximate amount to induce muscle building (hypertrophy).

6. Breathing is important. Don't hold your breath. Normally, you should exhale on the exertion phase of most exercises. For example, when doing a bench press, exhale once your arms are fully extended, then inhale as you lower your arms. Rest approximately 60-90 seconds between each set. Move the weight slow and smooth without snapping your joints.

7. <u>Note to beginners</u>: Start with one or two sets for the first two weeks to get your body accustomed to the routines. It is not uncommon to have DOMS (Delayed Onset of Muscle Soreness). Minor muscular soreness is to be expected but should disappear after a few days. Your muscles need to get used to being stressed and this minor pain is actually a signal that your muscle fibers are being worked hard enough to achieve hypertrophy.

Please also note that Dead Lifts (Day 5 lower body) require a different breathing technique than other exercises. For this exercise, fill your lungs with air, do not round your back, and hold your breath as you finish lowering the weight, then exhale. This will protect your spine. It is highly recommended beginners receive professional instruction, particularly with this exercise.

8. What about stretching? Stretching is basic to increasing range of motion, takes several forms and has pros and cons. The three basic forms are static, dynamic and PNF (Proprioceptive Neuromuscular Facilitation). Static stretching is just as it implies: a muscle is placed under tension and maintained for a period of time (about 20 seconds). For example, stand erect, try to touch your toes and maintain this position for a few seconds. Dynamic stretching is free-flowing and more reflective of natural movement. Letting your arms twist freely around your torso is one example. PNF requires the assistance of a partner to help increase the tension on a muscle while it is being passively stretched.

Static stretching should only be done after you are very warm. I prefer to use this method after my workout. Performing static stretches before engaging in sports activity can reduce performance and increase the risk of injury. Dynamic stretching is more appropriate to use before sports activity since it does not take you out of your normal range of motion, which can occur during a static stretch. PNF is effective in increasing range of motion, but should only be done with a qualified trainer or therapist. One other form of stretching, ballistic, e.g. bouncing movements, should only be used after a full warm up, and like static stretching, should not be used before an athletic event.

Some trainers swear by static stretching, but my advice is to play it on the safe side and use dynamic movements whenever possible. Static stretching may improve ROM (range of motion) and even blood flow, but there are other factors affecting ROM (joint configuration, soft tissue composition, collagen elasticity and scar tissue). To be safe, wait until you are done with all your activities before using the static method.

3 DAY STRENGTH TRAINING ROUTINE

	Sets	Repetition
DAY 1 (Arms, Biceps & Abdominals)		
1. Dumbbell Chest Press	3	10
2. Dumbbell Bicep Curls	3	10
3. Pec Flys	3	10
4. Dumbbell Hammer Curls	3	10
5. Push ups	3	10
6. Incline Machine Chest Press	3	10
7. Stability Ball Crunches	3	12
8. Russian Twist	3	12
9. Oblique Side Bends	3	12
10. Lying Hamstring Stretch	1	20 seconds each leg
11. Lying Glute Stretch	1	20 seconds each leg
DAY 3 (Shoulder, Back, Triceps & Abdominals)		
1. Seated Overhead Shoulder Press	3	10
2. Lat Pulldown	3	10
3. Seated Cable Row	3	10
4. Triceps Rope Pull Down	3	10
5. Lateral Raise	3	10
6. Front Raise	3	10
7. Rear Deltoid Raise	3	10
8. Overhead Triceps Extension	3	10
9. Abdominals	(repeat Day 1, exercises #7-11)	

	Sets	Repetition
DAY 5 (Lower Body & Abdominals)		
1. Stability Ball Prisoner squats	3	10
2. Walking Lunge w/twist	3	10
3. Seated Leg Press (Hack Squat)	3	10
4. Back extension (aka back raise)	3	10
5. Seated Hip Abduction	3	10
6. Seated Hip Adduction	3	10
7. Standing Calf Raise	3	10
8. Bent leg Dead Lift	3	15
9. Abdominals	(repeat day 1, exercises #7-11)	

Adjustments for Intermediate and Advanced Workouts:
There are many options for more advanced workouts. One is to alternate every week changing the number of sets and repetitions. For example, after a week of doing three sets of 10 repetitions, switch to two to six sets of four to six repetitions (this will require using heavier weights). In the following week, switch to three sets of 20 repetitions and use lighter weights. This should enable you to make additional gains in both strength and endurance and is one of numerous program designs which can be used to increase endurance, strength and power.

The exercises listed in this plan are designed for overall muscular balance. These pushing, pulling, pressing upward, squatting and twisting exercises are all basic movements and when performed correctly will produce excellent functional results. Begin with a competent certified personal trainer to ensure you are performing the exercises properly and to account for any individual differences of age, body type and physical condition.

DAY 1 (Biceps, Chest & Abdominals)

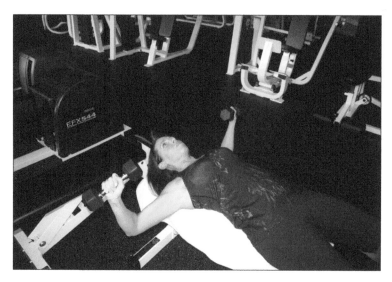

1. Dumbbell Chest Press (Starting Position)

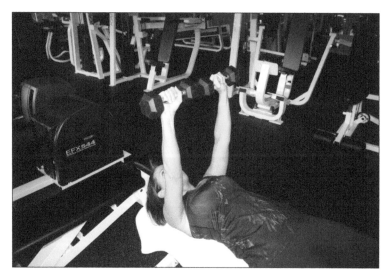

1. Dumbbell Chest Press (Finishing Position)

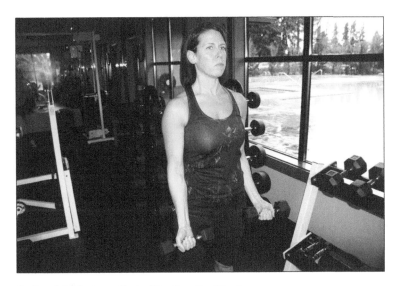

2. Dumbbell Bicep Curls (Starting Position)

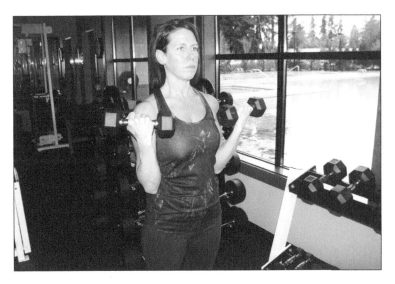

2. Dumbbell Bicep Curls (Finishing Position)

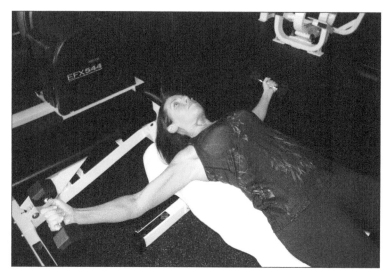

3. Pec Flys (Starting Position)

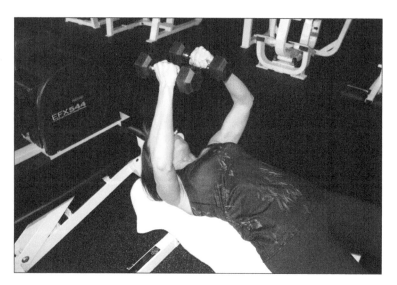

3. Pec Flys (Finishing Position)

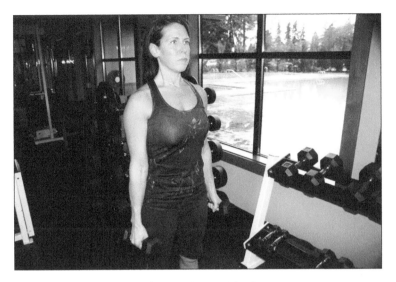

4. Dumbbell Hammer Curls (Starting Position)

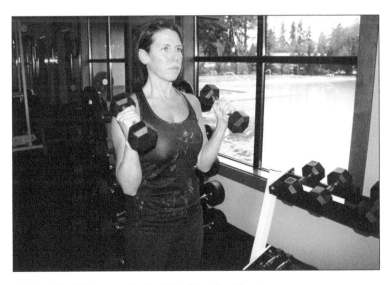

4. Dumbbell Hammer Curls (Finishing Position)

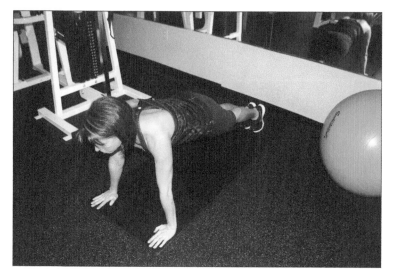

5. Push Ups (Starting Position)

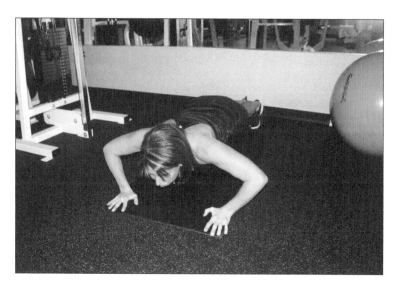

5. Push Ups (Finishing Position)

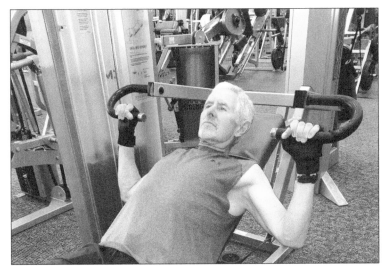

6. Incline Machine Chest Press (Starting Position)

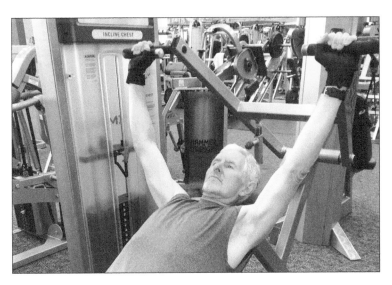

6. Incline Machine Chest Press (Finishing Position)

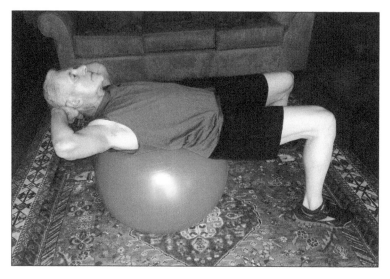

7. Stability Ball Crunches (Starting Position)

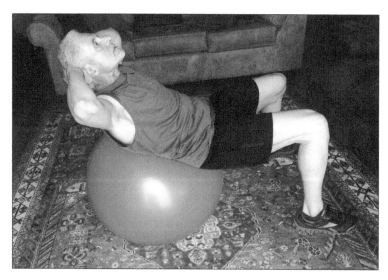

7. Stability Ball Crunches (Finishing Position)

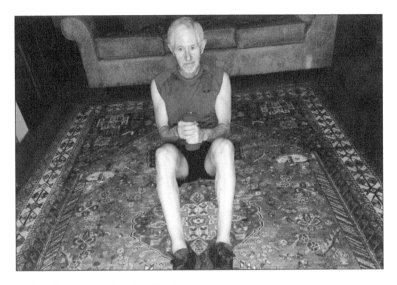

8. Russian Twist (Starting Position)

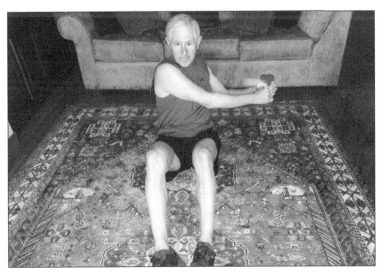

8. Russian Twist (First movement: then twist in opposite direction for finishing position)

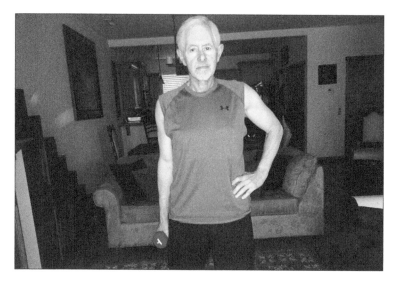

9. Oblique Side Bends (Starting Position)

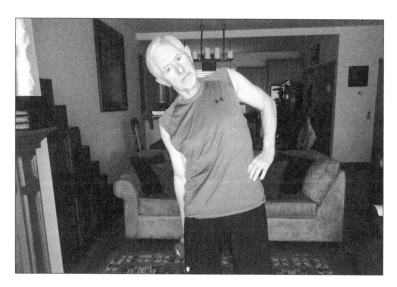

9. Oblique Side Bends (Finishing Position: then switch hands and
   repeat movement)

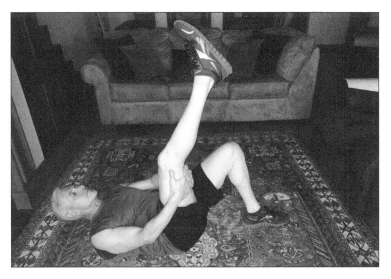

10. Hamstring Stretch (20 second hold, each leg)

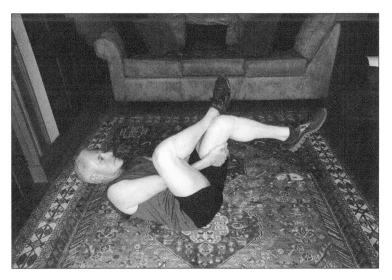

11. Glute Stretch (20 second hold, each leg)

DAY 3 (Shoulders, back, triceps & abdominals)

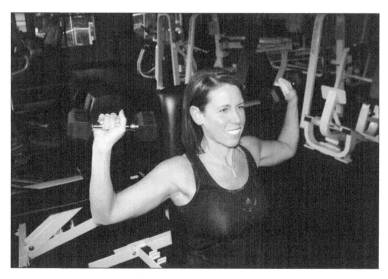

1. Seated Overhead Shoulder Press (Starting Position)

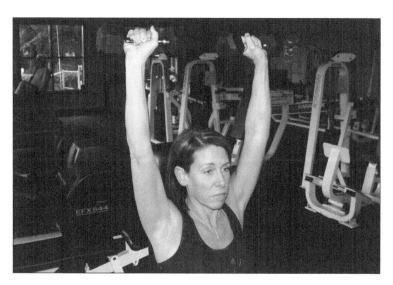

1. Seated Overhead Shoulder Press (Finishing Position)

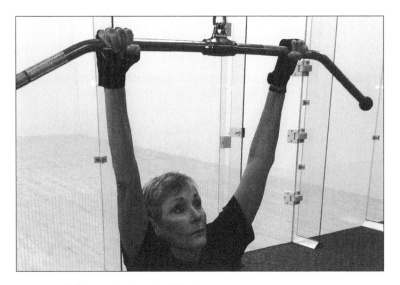

2. Lat Pull down (Starting Position)

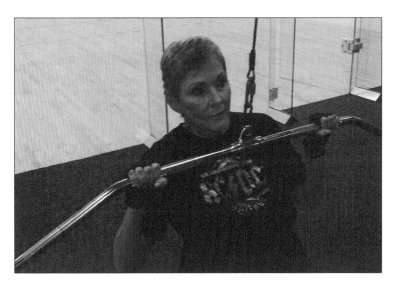

2. Lat Pull down (Finishing Position)

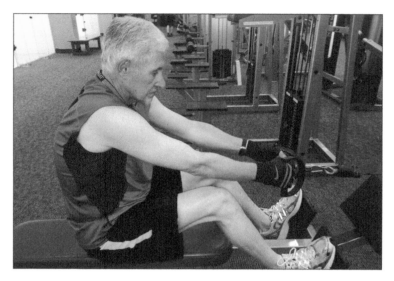

3. Seated Cable Row (Starting Position)

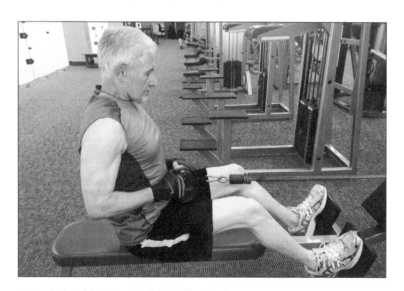

3. Seated Cable Row (Finishing Position)

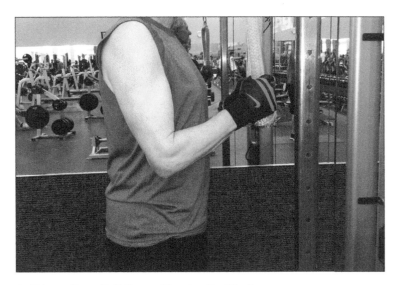

4. Triceps Rope Pull Down (Starting Position)

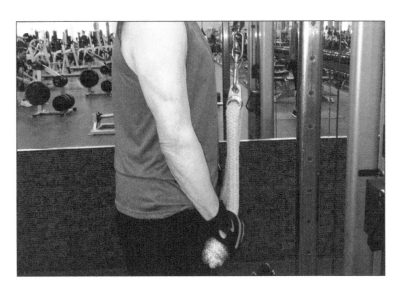

4. Triceps Rope Pull Down (Finishing Position)

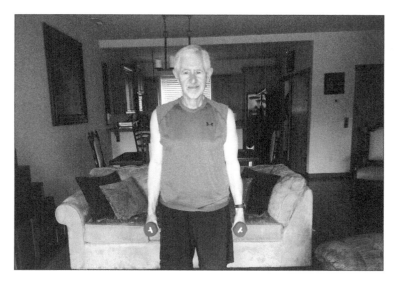

5. Lateral Raise (Starting Position)

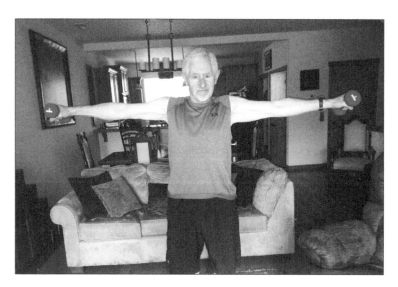

5. Lateral Raise (Finishing Position)

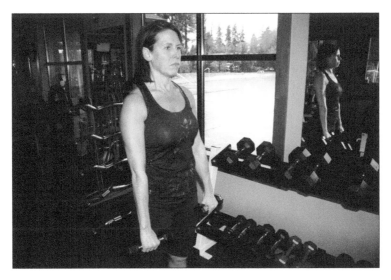

6. Alternating Front Raise (Starting Position)

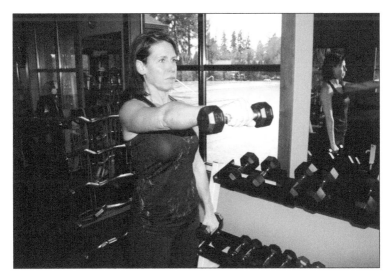

6. Alternating Front Raise (Alternate arm to finish one rep)

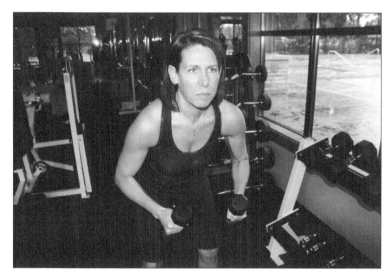

7. Rear Deltoid Raise (Starting Position)

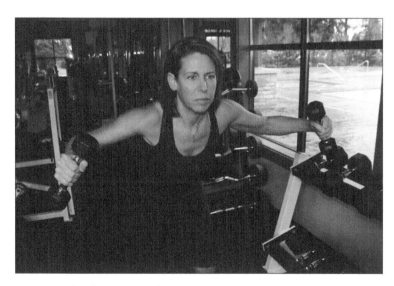

7. Rear Deltoid Raise (Finishing Position)

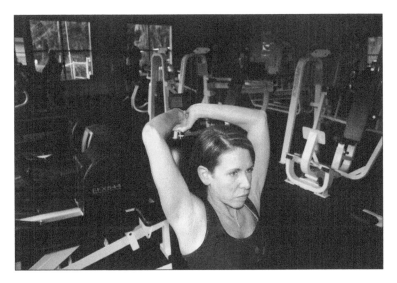

8. Overhead Dumbbell Triceps Extension (Starting Position)

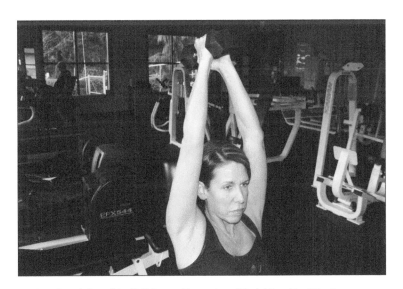

8. Overhead Dumbbell Triceps Extension (Finishing Position)

9. For abdominals and stretches, repeat Day 1 exercises #7-11

DAY 5 (Lower Body, Abdominals & Stretches)

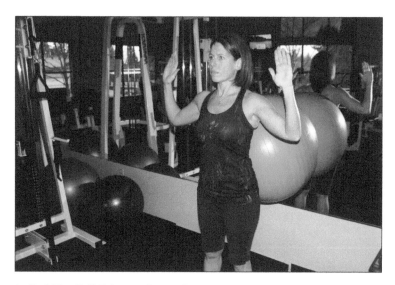

1. Stability Ball Prisoner Squat (Starting Position)

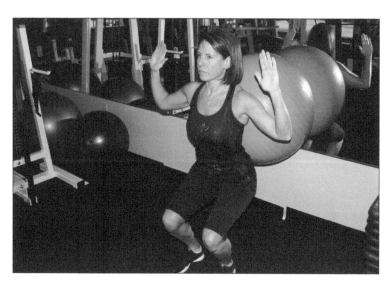

1. Stability Ball Prisoner Squat (Finishing Position)

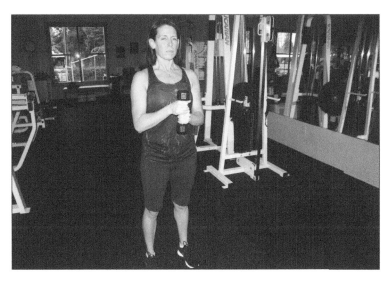

2. Walking Lunge with Twist (Starting Position)

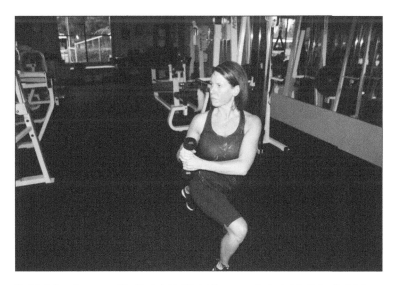

2. Walking Lunge with Twist (Initial Movement: twist left to finish)

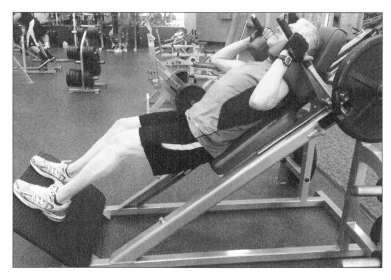

3. Hack Squat Machine (Starting Position)

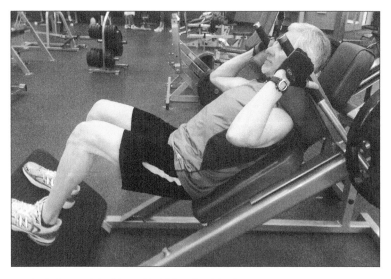

3. Hack Squat Machine (Finishing Position)

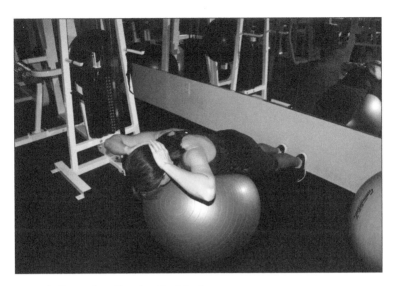

4. Back Extension (Starting Position)

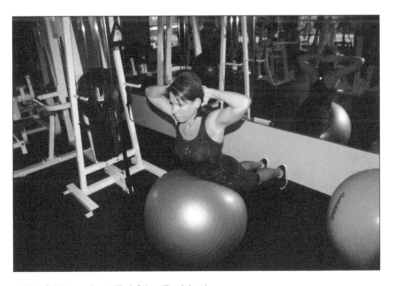

4. Back Extension (Finishing Position)

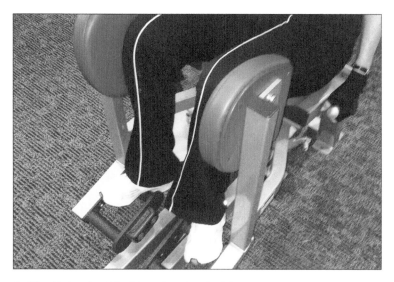

5. Hip Abduction Machine (Starting Position)

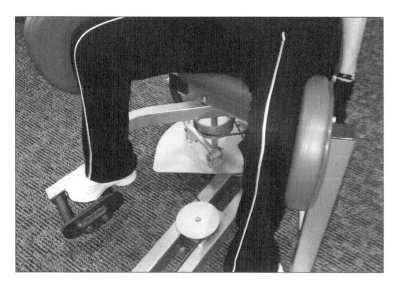

5. Hip Abduction Machine (Finishing Position)

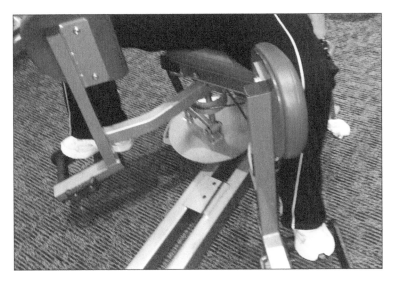

6. Hip Adduction Machine (Starting Position)

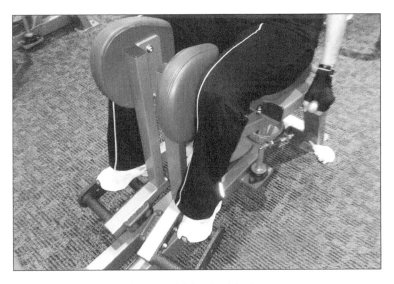

6. Hip Adduction Machine (Finishing Position)

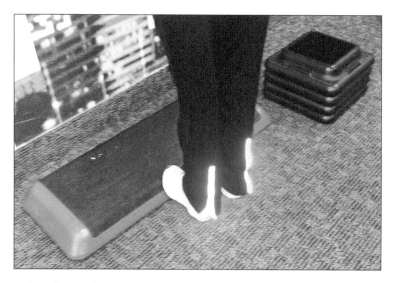

7. Standing Body Weight Calf Raise (Starting Position)

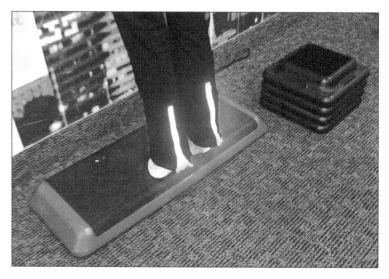

7. Standing Body Weight Calf Raise (Finishing Position)

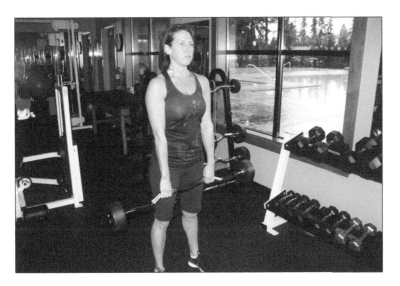

8. Bent Leg Dead Lift (Starting Position)

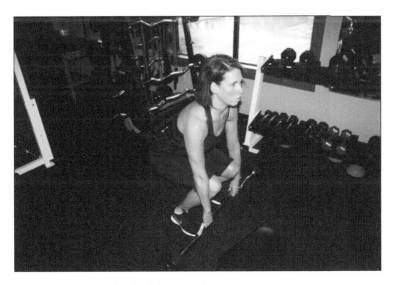

8. Bent Leg Dead Lift (Finishing Position)
9. For abdominals and stretches, repeat Day 1 exercises #7-11

CHAPTER 8

SHORT TAKES

VITAMINS & SUPPLEMENTS

The use of vitamins and supplements is a subject of ongoing discussion. There are no regulatory agencies administering to supplement manufacturers as the FDA does with prescription drugs. Therefore, we are all subject to variations in quality and the claims made by those marketing these products. I am hopeful that soon, most if not all marketed supplements will get some type of regulatory oversight.

As a general rule, vitamins are prevalent in the foods we eat and if we consume a wide variety of fruits, vegetables and good sources of protein we would in theory not need supplements. We are all genetically a bit different and there is no one diet that fits all. Since most unpackaged products do not come with the vitamin or mineral content pasted on them, it's difficult to know if we are getting all the nutrients we need to keep our metabolism and immune system in proper working order. Most doctors prescribe vitamins and minerals based on blood tests, age and other factors. Yet, even physicians admit there's not much scientific data on many supplements. The world of marketing, however, has tried to convince us we need all kinds of herbs, roots, minerals and other compounds to live a healthy life or to cure chronic disease. The school is still out on this subject.

I am going to share with you my personal experience on supplements, what I take as a senior, and why I take them. While my personal physician is on board with these, he freely admits there's not a lot of clinical data to support their usage. What I try to look for is any published data on toxicity, side effects, or detrimental outcomes of long term use. So here goes:

COLOSTRUM

Colostrum is the milk-like substance generated in the first few seconds of breastfeeding. It contains antibodies to protect newborn babies against disease during the first few months of life. It is high in protein and immune factors. Colostrum (made from bovine sources) has notably been taken for years by Olympic Athletes to prevent colds, build immune systems, and aid in the recovery after the stress of workouts. I have been using this substance for 8 years now (in pill form) and during this time I've had just two colds each of which lasted for only 3 days. I take 800 mg each morning on an empty stomach. I have not had any side effects. Anyone who is lactose intolerant, however, should not take this product without approval from a physician.

I am a big fan of colostrum as a dietary supplement and believe its application would benefit many in bolstering their immune system. With antioxidant compounds such as hemopexin and lactoferrin and rich in immune factors, I can't see any downsides to using colostrum as indicated unless you are lactose intolerant or have some other type of allergic response.

GLUCOSAMINE

This substance is normally found in the body, but natural levels seem to decline as we age. Supplements have been used in the treatment of arthritis and for minor joint pain. I have been taking 1500 mg in pill form (one in the morning and one in the evening). The product also contains 3.3 mg of Hyaluronic Acid (a joint lubricant) and 400 IU's of Vitamin D3 (necessary for the regulation of body minerals, bone health, immune system support and many other critical body functions).

Side effects reported have been generally mild, but there is not much research data on exactly how this product works. At an April 2014 conference I attended on aging, a physician reported that perhaps Glucosamine works more like a natural pain reliever than by actually lubricating joints. I have been using this as a supplement for several years and without it I notice stiffness and some shoulder pain, particularly in the morning. Taking it regularly has eliminated the pain and stiffness, so I plan to continue using it.

ASPIRIN

My family has a history of heart disease so I have been taking an 81 mg enteric coated aspirin for the past 10 years. So far I have had no side effects. A May 2014 FDA report announced taking daily low doses of aspirin were not recommended for healthy people since their data suggests the risk of heart attack is outweighed by the risk of bleeding. [15]

Daily regular dose (325 mg) and low dose (81mg) aspirin have been compared in several clinical trials for their effect on cardiovascular disease and stroke. In terms of efficacy, there appears to be no difference with the higher dose. Bleeding risk, however, *is* increased with the higher dose.[15] My advice is if you are one of the millions of Americans taking aspirin on a regular basis you should review this practice with your physician. There are some who don't agree with the FDA, so you should discuss this issue with your personal physician.

FISH OIL

I take 1400 mg per day of fish oil as a supplement, but skip it on days when I eat fish. If you eat fish more than twice a week, you may not need to supplement with fish oil. While there's quite some evidence that the Omega-3's in the fish oil support heart health by lowering triglycerides, taking too much in the way of supplements may have the opposite effect. Again, it is wise to consult your physician before popping these Omega-3 bombs.

METABOLIC SYNDROME

This condition is associated with obesity and characterized by high blood pressure, high fasting blood sugar and high cholesterol levels, all of which are unwanted health threats. Having these markers greatly increase the risk of acquiring cardiovascular disease, diabetes, cancer or any combination thereof and, along with the misery factor of acquiring them, they will almost certainly shorten your life. If you happen to fall in this category or are headed in this direction, it would be wise to diligently and quickly follow the instructions contained in the preceding chapters.

One thing I have learned about this syndrome, as with smoking, the habits which have led to this condition are hard to kick. A consistently poor diet and a sedentary lifestyle are not just acquired by osmosis. These are habits developed over years and have both physical and/or psychological origin. Food, especially those high in refined sugar, and nicotine addictions are tough to beat. Victory over these dangerous habits takes determination and support. Some people can do it alone, others need help. Weight loss and smoking clinics throughout the country specialize in these issues. Success rates vary to be sure, but the habits can be kicked.

You and I can walk in any mall and easily see the signs of metabolic syndrome. It's epidemic. The fix is no different than maintaining your car. You've got to have the right fuel (a proper diet) and perform routine maintenance (aerobic and anaerobic exercise) to keep the machine below your brain (your body) working properly. If you happen to think, as many smoking and food addicts do, that there's plenty of time to quit before any harm is done, think again.

FOR GOLFERS

Golf is one of the few sports that can be played at almost any age. Many have criticized golf for not being a "real" sport (although a recent Costco poll shows 59 percent think it is). As a TPI (Titleist Performance Institute) Certified Golf Fitness Instructor, I can tell you with certainty that golf requires an array of skills sets and physical attributes including joint mobility and stability, which is why fitness training for golf has undergone a major revolution.

Golf requires both aerobic and anaerobic fitness, coordination and balance, a solid mental approach and like any other sport—practice. The Champions Tour, for professionals over the age of 50, proves senior players can play the game at a very high level. Many seniors can compete on the regular PGA tour although they are at some disadvantage against the younger tour players who are hitting the ball longer than previously thought possible. Physical training and equipment technology are both responsible, but regardless of age the fact is that being fit has a lot to do with finishing a round of golf without fatigue. My advice, if you are able, is to leave the power cart behind and walk the course. You won't build endurance or burn calories by sitting on your butt. If you have a disability or injury, however, taking a cart will still allow you to have fun.

If it were up to me, golf would be a required subject in grade schools. It teaches so much more than the sport is given credit for including patience, discipline, honesty, mental focus and physical fitness. In my view, if golf education were required around the world, many of our social problems would be reduced significantly. Golf teaches a universal language beyond the spirit of competition while being played in an open air "green" environment. While there are downsides (it's time consuming, expensive for many, and can be frustrating to those whose personalities are not attuned to the constant changing conditions and the practice necessary to have some mastery of the game), the upsides are too vast to ignore.

My experience working with foster children in both the First Tee program in Portland, OR and now with the Summit Golf Foundation (www.Summitgolf.org), has proven that well designed youth golf programs can improve self-esteem while emphasizing education, diversity, positive character traits and the management of adversity. While the sport does not appeal to everyone, golf has a lot to offer.

Whether you're nine or ninety, golf is a game that individuals, groups and families can enjoy. It is soon to become an Olympic event because it is recognized around the world for its high degree of competition, honor and fair play, Add wind, sand traps, water hazards and undulating greens and, the truth be told—the real competition in golf is between the player and the course. This indeed makes it seem like it's not a sport after all, rather a never ending battle with Mother Nature herself.

Sometimes, just watching the face of kid who has sunk a long putt is enough for me, but seeing a foster child using his or her golf experience to overcome life's obstacles and become motivated to finish school is about as good as it can get.

FOR RUNNERS: A WORD TO THE WISE

If you're a regular runner then it's likely your heart and lung function is in good shape. Depending on how long you run and the level of effort expended, your body is using oxygen more efficiently and you're probably able to manage your weight. If you have not lost any pounds, or if you have gained weight with your running program, then look to your diet for the cause and adjust accordingly.

Even if you are happy with your current running program and you like all the positive things you've achieved, there can be some serious long term downsides. While running is one of the best all-around cardiovascular exercises, it can have detrimental effects on your bones and joints. Long-term runners who make it to their 60s, 70s and beyond often suffer from knee and hip injuries. Certainly body types and genetics play a role in how much wear and tear hips, knees, feet and back can take, but I have seen too many older runners who have chronic knee, hip, back and foot pain as a result of a long-term running program. Orthopedic surgeons are thriving on all the baby boomers who took up running as the answer to improving their metabolic health and managing their weight. These individuals have likely avoided heart attack and stroke, but now face structural issues, pain and immobility. So what's the answer?

Many aerobic options are lower in impact and have all the benefits of running without the pounding and risk of injury. While some are already using treadmills (a bit better option than running on pavement), the best way to avoid these injuries is to switch to lower impact training such as elliptical trainers or the recumbent or traditional bicycles. These lower impact aerobic activities can burn just as many calories and condition your heart and lungs without the detrimental effects of high impact running. If you have reached your 40s without any serious injury to your knees or hips, I suggest you consider reducing your running program and transition to lower impact activities. There is also evidence that pushing your body too hard for too long can have an adverse cardiovascular effect. More research is needed in this area, but this does makes sense. It's not unlike consistently running your car at a very high RPM. Perhaps our bodies should also have a red line.

FOR SENIORS

Having trained many seniors (and being one myself), I know adopting new and strenuous activities later in life can be problematic. It takes desire, determination and mental discipline to make changes to a long-standing sedentary lifestyle. Poor dietary and exercise habits that have existed for decades can create the conditions for obesity, lack of energy, frailty and depression. I see it all the time. It saddens me when people in their 70s or 80s come to me for help after leading sedentary lifestyles for many years. They may be alive, but they are not enjoying the golden years they were promised, even if their finances are sound. All the cash in the world or having the best health insurance will not make a difference if your body has decayed through years of neglect.

Cancer, cardiovascular disease, arthritis, osteoporosis, diabetes and frailty are commonplace among the aged. While diet and exercise alone may not be the exclusive answer to avoiding these diseases, in most cases they are the best form of insurance you can buy. Metabolic fitness, when your body uses fuel in the form of fat and carbohydrates in the most efficient manner, will not just help protect you from these unwanted maladies, but will give you both a mental and physical advantage as you age. You will feel more energetic and vital with enough strength to climb those stairs or even mountains. Many of my older clients are doing this every day and it is wonderful to see them thrive.

For those who would like more specifics about living longer and in good health, one of the best books I know is "Biomarkers" by William Evans, Ph.D. and Irwin H Rosenberg, M.D. This book describes the metabolic factors of aging and offers a detailed prescription for maintaining vitality. It's based on research from the USDA Human Research Center on Aging at Tufts University.

A serious issue plaguing seniors is their propensity to fall and sustain serious injury or die due to a decline in proprioception (the perception of where one's body is in space). Impaired reaction times, poor vision and vestibular functions can create the perfect storm for falls. While these issues are complex and involve several human physiological functions, sensor-motor functional assessment is important to diagnose balance issues in older adults. Finding the right modalities for these age-related changes is an ongoing process.

In a 2007 study, researchers S.W. Shaffer and A.L. Harrison concluded there is need to provide some older adults with "compensatory strategies that increase sensory information during function" as well as "interventions designed to enhance recovery of sensory and balance function." Their study pointed to the need to distinguish between the young-old and old-old adult populations when developing intervention strategies. They concluded the younger group needed to focus on enhancing function while the older group should focus on compensation strategies e.g., visually marking boundaries like curbs and steps. [17]

I have seen the results of weight and balance training in older adults that improve their strength and agility to help them avoid falls. Most physical therapists today have a wide range of evaluative tools to identify motor and muscular issues that can affect balance as well as a number of exercises and drills to improve posture and stability. In this regard I am a big fan of using ankle and wrist weights to provide lower extremity sensory feedback. Many fitness centers are now addressing balance issues, but for older adults with high risks of falling, I suggest a physical therapist or fitness trainer who can perform the appropriate balance tests and prescribe an appropriate course of action.

It is troublesome that so much misinformation abounds in both the printed and digital world. Do this, do that, try this, try that are often just simple marketing tools cleverly disguised to take your money. If your neighbor swears eating porcupine needles all his life has kept him alive, and he's 90 years old and in good health, perhaps it seems logical to follow the same path. So much is clouded in superstition, old wives tales, opinions and marketing gimmicks it is hard to separate sense from nonsense. So where's the truth?

Follow the old rule—if it sounds too good to be true, it probably is. Ask questions, lots of them. Remember, what may work for your friend or neighbor may not work for you and can even be harmful. Spend time checking things out before you decide on accepting a non-professional opinion on diet or exercise. The truth is sometimes hard to find, but it's out there. You may not always like the answer, but at least you will have done your homework and perhaps saved yourself some grief and considerable expense.

FOR WALKERS

You've probably read or heard how good walking is for your health, especially for seniors. If walking is exercise, however, then is changing the oil in your car the only maintenance it needs? Of course not! Walking is not exercise! It's *an* exercise, just one of many exercises you need to maintain your health and fitness.

I often get new clients who tell me they walk five or more miles a day. I always congratulate them on this very important activity, but at the same time tell them I have serious doubts walking by itself will do much to insure they live longer, unless you compare this to not walking at all and then this is probably true. Why is this so?

For the most part, unless you walk very fast and keep your heart rate consistently high, walking does not produce enough stress for the body to adapt to a higher metabolic level. While it's likely to keep your joints lubricated and your muscles activated, it does not do much to protect against sarcopenia (age related loss of muscle mass). Also, to produce any significant improvement to your heart or lungs, you must walk fast enough to get your heart rate to a level that will cause positive adaptation to your cardiovascular system (normally between 55 percent to 85 percent of your heart rate maximum). Therefore, I always recommend using a heart rate monitor when walking.

Certainly walking will burn some needed calories and that's a good thing, so don't stop. To effectively care for your body, however, you need to have a more complete program that includes strength training. For those of you who diet from time to time, beware!! Dieting may bring weight loss but it also brings muscle loss. If you don't replace the muscle loss through strength training, you will become weaker and eventually frail. This normally doesn't become a concern until you're older, but then it can become a very big problem. Without practicing strength training, many seniors can't even make it up a small flight of stairs.

HOODIES: NOT FOR THE GYM

Every generation has its fashion markers and it seems today "hoodies" are in style. The good thing about them is they seem to do a good job of keeping your head warm, but they have absolutely no place in the gym environment. In fact, they're downright dangerous.

Your body has basically two ways to protect its cells: fat and water. If you wear a hoodie while working out, your body temperature will rise and you'll begin to sweat (the body's way of cooling you). The hoodie, however, will trap the heat and not allow the sweat to do its job. Then as your body temperature rises, your heart will do what it's designed to do in these situations and that's to pump faster. Because you're generating more heat you'll begin to get dehydrated. So now you have two problems. Your heart is working a lot harder than it should and your body, trying to protect its cells, will hold on to fat like a duck holding on to a June bug. Not only won't you lose weight, you may put your heart, kidneys and muscles at risk.

It seems many people still believe sweating it out in the gym will help them lose weight. In fact, all sweating does is make you lose water weight and that's downright danger-ous—at any age. Young people who push themselves too hard and sweat too much may experience breakdown of muscle tissue (rhabdomyolysis) and/or renal failure. Older folks wearing hoodies could have a heart attack or stroke, especially if they have any underlying medical conditions. The bottom line is wearing a hoodie is great if you want to stay warm, but as workout apparel goes it's a bad move. Leave it in your locker.

SOME FACTS ABOUT PLANT-BASED DIETS

Plant-based diets have become popular over the past few years. "Vegetarian" diets (which primarily contain foods of plant origin) and "Vegan" diets (only from the plant king-dom having no animal product ingredients) are believed by many to be healthier alternatives to diets that allow meat and are better for the environment.

While a significant portion of the world's annual grain harvest goes to feed farm animals, and reducing meat consumption would likely be beneficial, there are some important physiological issues to consider before totally giving up meat in your diet. Meat is not only a significant source of protein, but it contains important vitamins and minerals needed by the body. For example:

- Vitamin B12 is produced by bacterial fermentation and found primarily in animal products. Supplementation with this vitamin may be critical in a vegetarian/vegan diet.
- Calcium is found in many green leafy vegetables, however, some compounds found in a plant-only diet can hinder calcium absorption. Again, supplementation may be necessary.
- Omega-3 fatty acids are important to prevent certain diseases and play a role in body composition. People on plant-based diets can have lower blood concentrations of these acids than meat eaters. While flax, walnuts and canola do contain Omega-3's, supplements may need to be considered.
- Vitamin D is not found in many plant foods. Supplements and additional amounts of sunlight may be necessary.
- Soy is a major source of proteins in plant-based diets. Large amounts of soy intake may affect thyroid function if iodine intake is limited. Iodized or sea salt may be necessary in these diets.

While going vegetarian or vegan is a personal choice, it is wise to consult with your physician and/or nutrition professional before entirely eliminating meats. The health benefits of a plant-based diet can still be achieved by reducing the intake of animal protein and increasing the percentage of fruits, vegetables, nuts, legumes and seeds. Consider all your options before adopting a strict vegetarian or vegan diet.

GUIDELINES FOR PRE-TEENS

Complexities abound with pre-teen metabolism and growth. Children not only grow at different rates compared to others, but their body parts may grow at different rates as well. Some mature early and some late. Managing growth spurts is not just a science but often an art form.

Because children differ in growth behavior, and have varying metabolic profiles, parents need to closely observe their child's growth rate and behavior. Poor dietary choices and lack of exercise can spiral out of control due to unwanted physical and/or emotional changes. Additionally, not all children have access to parks and other recreational environments. Weather also poses challenges to outside activities. To overcome these obstacles and give children the best possible metabolic and developmental advantages, I offer the following guidelines:

- Make sure your child has regular medical evaluations by a physician who specializes in child development. Do not change diets without consulting your medical provider.
- Most exercise for pre-teens should take the form of play: running, jumping, hopping, skipping, climbing (with restrictions and supervision), and engaging in a variety of physical exertion activities. This helps to develop aerobic capacity as well as motor and coordination skills.
- See that your child gets adequate amounts of sleep and rest.
- Offer a balanced diet with plenty of fresh fruits and vegetables, lean sources of protein with limited amounts of processed sugars, sodium and saturated fat.

- Make sure your child is adequately hydrated, especially when playing and engaging in sports.
- For those who are keen on specialty sports (like golf or tennis), practice time is valuable. Other forms of exercise, however, should be included to balance a child's developmental skills.
- Emphasize and encourage scholastic excellence.
- Managing weight during this phase of growth is problematic. Growth and exercise increase hunger so children need proper nutrients to insure structural growth and development. Track your child's Body Mass Index (BMI) on a regular basis (refer to the Calculating your BMI table in Chapter 6).
- Weight training per se is not normally recommended for pre-teens since most growth and development is initiated by hormonal changes.

PERSONAL TRAINING

The criteria for selecting a certified personal trainer are similar to choosing other professional services. Professionalism, education, experience, proven results and trusted referrals are all positive indicators. The question you may ask, however, is why do I need one at all? Can't I just buy a video, use an app, or follow written instructions?

Certainly it is a more expensive option to workout with a personal trainer, but consider the following before you decide to go it on your own. A trainer can help you avoid both simple and potentially costly mistakes. A good trainer will evaluate your physical condition and develop a plan that is specific to you. He, or she, will teach you the proper form to avoid injury, give you varying routines to improve results, and make sure you don't develop planar imbalances that can lead to pain and loss of functionality.

One of the biggest faux pas I see by those who train themselves is they read a magazine or visit a website, and they follow a workout designed for a professional athlete. What's good for them must be good for me, right? Many times these routines are only a snapshot of what the pro actually does and more than likely these routines require a very high level of fitness with months of practice. This can easily lead an amateur down a path to serious injury or muscular imbalance.

Effective personal training takes proper assessment before beginning any workout program. It can only have value if it accomplishes your desired goals e.g. improved strength, flexibility, weight loss, etc., and does so safely. Going it on your own is risky. I have seen too many "gym rats" who look like they know what they're doing, but have major muscle imbalances (and pain) because they don't really know what muscles (and groups of muscles) to train and in the proper proportion. Consider these questions: How much work do my abs need? How often do I work my traps, glutes, hamstrings, quads, biceps, triceps, lats, deltoids, pecs, etc? What's the proper level of resistance? Which exercises are the most effective? What kind of stretches do I need? What about dietary requirements and hydration? Professional trainers can answer these questions knowledgeably and provide specific programs and instruction so you can avoid the pitfalls of muscular imbalances, over/under training, not to mention injury and pain.

So where do you find the best trainers? If you don't have a friend or relative who can give you a solid referral, then please go the Resources section at the end of this book that will give you some excellent websites to enable you to find one. Many of the larger fitness centers do have competent trainers, just make sure they have experience working with your age group and with any specific medical or physical condition you may have.

THE MAGIC OF MINDFULNESS

Despite all you can do to improve your health with proper diet and exercise protocols, another critical factor can make a huge difference in how well and how long you live. The space between our ears houses the "General" of our body with the control over our thoughts, emotions and behaviors that affect every part of us, including our health.

Life is a lot like baseball. You step up to the plate and you don't know if you're going to get a fastball, slider, sinker, change up, knuckle ball or curve ball. Will it be high or low? Inside or outside? Good hitters prepare both mentally and physically for any of them. Just as in baseball we know curves are coming; we just don't know when. The practice of mindfulness is a way to focus our thoughts to deal with the complexities and curve balls of the world.

For centuries several eastern religions have espoused meditation and self-reflection as a way to calm the mind, body and spirit. The practice of finding peace and tranquility, focusing on the present in a nonjudgmental way, and using reflective and awareness skills to modify behaviors is not just confined to religious dogma. It can apply to almost every human endeavor: sports, business, and/or personal relationships. The need for harmony in our daily life is often critical to how our body functions. The mind and body are one. The practice of yoga, for example, is but one of the many excellent pathways for including mindfulness in the process of maintaining our overall health and wellness.

Author Vivian Greene has said, "Life is not about waiting for the storm to pass, but learning how to dance in the rain!" Taking time to be meditative and reflective is a way to sort our thoughts and emotions and can be critical to establishing the homeostasis our physiology seeks. The resolution of inner conflict is a major outcome in the practice of mindfulness. While this skill may come naturally to some, for others it is more difficult yet worthwhile to pursue.

GOYA (GET OFF YOUR ASS)

You've just had an annual physical exam and your physician tells you everything "is" fine and dandy. Whew!! Another year of dodging a bullet! The problem, however, is your medical provider may not have fully explained the full significance of your exam. You see, what you've been told is not in the present tense.

This apparently small grammatical difference is most important in terms of your on-going health. Your physical exam represents only the past. It has nothing to do with what's going to happen in the future. Just because you were healthy yesterday or even today does not mean you will be healthy tomorrow. Health, I'm sure you'll agree, is much better if it's sustainable—day in, day out, week in, week out, year in, year out. For the most part being healthy takes the same process that keeps your car in proper running order and that my friends, is scheduled maintenance.

Your car requires regular oil changes, having the tires and brakes checked and other tests to determine key operating systems. For your body it means getting periodic medical checkups, eating the right foods, exercising regularly, and routinely watching some vital measurements—for starters: cholesterol levels, blood pressure, blood sugar level, bone density and body fat percentage.

So if you passed your last physical with flying colors, don't think for a minute it's a signal you are going to be healthy indefinitely. It's no different than having your picture taken. One second after it's taken you're a tad older and likely you will never look exactly like that again.

It is not precisely clear why many physicians do not explain this very simple yet highly important factoid to their patients. It may be they think it's too obvious, or perhaps it's not relevant in terms of their training, which is directed almost exclusively on trying to fix what ails you. After all, you wouldn't go to a doctor (other than for an annual physical) if nothing was wrong. Many family doctors and primary care physicians are not wellness directed. Their forte is the diagnosis and cure of disease and illness, and generally speaking, they don't give you a whole lot of wellness information (my sincere apologies and kudos to those physicians who do take the time and effort to communicate wellness information by counseling patients on proper diet and exercise).

Fitness and nutritional training have a very relevant place in the world of health. They not only supplement what your medical provider may prescribe for your individual health situation, but they provide the action pathway to prevent many age-related diseases by maintaining your body systems so they can perform as intended. Disease and frailty later in life, in many cases, are avoidable. You can increase your chance of living well into your 80s and even 90s with strength and vitality by managing all facets of your diet, exercising correctly on a regular basis, and using mindfulness to help manage the complexity of your thoughts and emotions. *This is not a guess. This is not myth. This is not marketing hype.* So GOYA!

FAQS

I want to get started on the DGOLF Diet plan, but how do I figure out how to eliminate 300 calories a day from my diet?

There are several ways to do this. One is to use a free app like *My Fitness Pal* to track your food intake. It has a feature that will tell you the caloric content of virtually every food along with the carbohydrate, protein and fat content. There are also many free websites that provide the caloric content of foods. One example is www.thecaloriecounter.com. Once you find the foods worth 300 calories (preferably those with high glycemic carbohydrates), eliminate them from your diet for four consecutive days as suggested in the DGOLF plan. What it takes is some pre-planning and a bit of discipline.

I'm not able to get to a fitness center. Do personal trainers make house calls?

Yes, check your local listings for at-home personal training. Virtually all cities and towns have trainers that will come to your home and help you with your fitness needs. It is always wise, however, to get a referral before you let anyone into your home. There are also several certifying organizations you can check with such as ACE (American Council on Exercise), NASM (National Academy of Sports Medicine) and ISSA (International Sports Sciences Association) that can tell you about certified trainers located in your area.

Re the workouts shown in Chapter 7, how long should I do them before they need to be updated?

The workouts shown in Chapter 7 are designed for beginners to build functional strength. Two to three months should get you on your way, and then transition to more advanced exercises. As time goes on, depending on your goals, you can increase weights and/or change intensities. Having a physical evaluation by a certified personal trainer is highly recommended to help you set proper goals and optimize your training conditions. Because everyone is a bit different in response to training, being monitored by a personal trainer is the best way to get superior results and avoid injury.

I can't afford a personal trainer and don't like lifting weights. Is there something else I can do?

The processes described in this book are designed to take advantage of proper diet, exercise and a positive mental approach to lower the risk of disease and slow the aging process. Some people convince themselves this approach is not necessary because they see others who live relatively healthy lives without any training or special dietary protocols. My advice is do what you can to expend physical energy on a daily basis. The human body was not designed to sit in front of a TV for months and years on end. Walk, use resistance bands (which are inexpensive), and do whatever you can to burn calories on a daily basis.

I'm disabled. What workouts can I do?

Being disabled is an opportunity to be creative. If you're confined to a wheel chair, you can still do most, if not all, of the upper body exercises shown in Chapter 7 as well as following the recommended low sugar, low saturated fat, nutrient-rich diet plan. If your lower body is restricted try to get assistance in moving your legs and/or massaging them on a daily basis or any other body part that is not mobile.

I've never worked out. What's the best way to get started?

Slowly. If you've never worked out before, or it's been a while, don't try to be a warrior. Take a few weeks and work on the aerobic side first. Walk to start, but transition to a faster pace when you feel comfortable. For weight training, you can start with resistance bands or light weights and then progress to more strenuous workouts. The secret is giving your body time to adapt to more strenuous levels of resistance. Two to three weeks of aerobic training then adding resistance for two to three weeks should get you ready to move forward to more advanced levels.

Should I expect muscle soreness when I workout?

Yes, some minor muscular pain should be expected. DOMS (Delayed Onset of Muscle Soreness) is actually a positive sign your muscles are adapting to the physical stress. Soreness should only last a few days, but it is almost an inevitable part of muscular adaptation. After a few workouts of each muscle group, they will adapt and soreness will no longer be an issue. If you change workouts, however, or take your muscles through a wider range of motion, you will again experience DOMS. Just remember it's actually a good sign your workouts are being effective!

Should I use machines or free weights?

Both can be used. The difference is machines are good at isolating muscles and keeping you in segment alignment. Therefore, machines are less likely to cause injury because the weight is more stable while free weights (like dumbbells, barbells and kettle bells) can be dropped or can shift and cause injury. Free weights have a training advantage because they require use of stabilizing muscles and are better for improving functional performance. Using free weights requires multiple muscle movements rather than isolating a muscle as machines do. Both have their place in training. I often recommend starting out with machines for beginners and transitioning to free weights. Even advanced athletes, however, use machines because they can focus on improving individual muscles and, when combined with other free weight exercises, do improve overall results. You'll notice the workout program featured in Chapter 7 makes use of both machines and free weights. The key to using free weights is getting the proper instruction to avoid injury.

How much sleep do I need?

Thousands of studies have been done on sleep and sleep deprivation. The best advice I can give you is to get as much sleep as you can at night. Some of your sleep habits are likely genetic, but emotional stress, diet, temperature, lighting conditions and hormonal balances can all affect the outcome of your night's rest. Given the variability and individual differences of human beings, one person may need five or six hours sleep and another 10 to feel rested, so there's not one answer. Sleep deprivation or disturbance can have significant impacts on our health and physical performance. If you feel tired because you suspect you're not getting enough sleep, then by all means, see your physician.

What about weight loss products like Raspberry Ketones and Garcinia Cambogia?

These products have been touted on TV as effective weight loss aides. Some people have had success using them, but there is only scant scientific research to validate the claims made by marketers. The American Journal of Weight Loss recently reported that Garcinia Cambogia had effective results in a weight loss study, "providing the grade of the product meets the standard." Again, manufacturers are unregulated and the quality of various brands, therefore, may be questionable. Consult your physician before using any of these products.

What about gluten-free?

A recent article by Consumer Reports® portrayed the gluten free craze to be mostly a marketing goldmine. Unless you have celiac disease or are otherwise allergic to wheat, barley or rye, this article indicated several possible downsides: 1) gluten free may not have as many vitamins or minerals, 2) gluten free may have a higher caloric content causing you weight gain, 3) some gluten-free products may be higher in arsenic content, 4) higher in price, and 5) perhaps five percent of gluten-free products don't meet the FDA's gluten-free guidelines. This could be a real problem for people with celiac disease.

Decide for yourself, but my suggestion is to always read the ingredients list and if you suspect you are allergic to gluten, get tested to make sure. Otherwise, you could be subject to the downsides as portrayed in this study ("The Truth About Gluten," Consumer Reports®, January 2015).

Are protein shakes a good source of energy?

Believe it or not, protein is not your body's choice for providing energy to your muscles. The majority of proteins are used to build and repair muscle tissue, bones, cartilage, and to construct hormones and enzymes. It is the body's last choice for use as muscular fuel. It is likely that most people are consuming too much protein. After the body is done breaking down proteins into amino acids and using them as described above, the remainder will either be discarded in your urine or converted to fat for storage. Ingesting too many proteins will force your body to use calcium and water to excrete the excess, so if you engage in sporting activities this can have a negative impact on hydration and central nervous system response (calcium ions are necessary for central nervous system function). If your activity is limited to changing TV channels with your remote, you probably won't feel any different by consuming too much protein, but long term there could be a detrimental effect on kidney function. So what's a proper amount? Accepted daily intake ranges are about .8 grams of protein per kilogram of body weight for non-athletes, somewhat higher for athletes depending on the sport (1.2-1.7 grams per kilogram of body weight).

What about so called Hypo-Oxic Training (oxygen deprivation)? Does it work and should I try it?

This training practice seems to be growing in popularity. Some fitness centers are even adding rooms that simulate high altitudes to offer training in an "oxygen deprived" environment. The theory is that depriving the body of oxygen will cause adaptive response and the body will use oxygen more efficiently and even increase red blood cells. There are also masks you can buy that similarly restrict oxygen intake. The body adapts to a variety of conditions, so in theory, this type of training makes some sense. Given that you can't perform as well or as long when deprived of oxygen, however, it begs the question whether this offsets the benefits of the deprivation. Some swear by it, but school is still out on how effective it really is. Based on the reality of individual differences, I would expect varying results. The other factor is safety. Younger athletes are certainly less likely to have negative results than older adults who may not be conditioned or may have some underlying medical condition that could spark a catastrophic series of events. If you do try it, make absolutely sure you have proper supervision.

ADDITIONAL RESOURCES

www.EXRX.net
A website with comprehensive resources for fitness assessment and instruction

www.Wikepedia.org
Reference Mindfulness: for definitions, history, practice and research; contains links to other mindfulness references and websites

www.GOL-FIT.com
My business website featuring golf-centric information, diet and nutrition, workouts, plus corporate and customized programs to help your health and your golf game

www.Summitgolf.org
A website devoted to helping young people excel in life through the game of golf

www.garytaubes.com
Author website with articles on diet, nutrition and health issues

www.issaonline.edu
International Sports Sciences Association website; specialists in educating and certifying personal trainers

Astrofit by Dr. William J. Evans
Book by noted author on anti-aging strategies based on diet
and nutritional protocols

APPENDIX

(ENDNOTES)

IN THE BEGINNING

1   McCarthy, Justin. "In U.S., Adult Obesity Rate Now at 27.7%." May 22, 2014. http://www.gallup.com

INTRODUCTION

2   U.S. Dept of Health and Human Services. *National Vital Statistics Report, United States Life Tables, Volume 59 Number 9 (2007).*

CHAPTER 2

3   Center for Disease Control and Prevention, National Center for Injury Prevention and Control. *Web-based Injury Statistics Query and Reporting System (WISQARS). Accessed August 15, 2013.*

4   Hatfield, Frederick C. 2004. *Fitness: The Complete Guide.* Carpinteria: International Sports Sciences Association.

5   Ibid.

CHAPTER 4

6   Ibid.

CHAPTER 5

7   Consumer Reports. 2014. *Food & Fitness* p 23-27.

8   Berardi, John, Phd. and Ryan Andrews.MS/ MA,RD.2009. Nutrition: The Complete Guide. Carpinteria: International Sports Sciences Association

9   Atkins, Robert C. M.D. 2003. *Atkins for Life*. New York: St. Martin's Press.

10 Davis, Lisa. "Is This Any Way to Lose Weight" *Reader's Digest*. Feb 2011. http://www.garytaubes.com

11 Evans, William, and Irwin H. Rosenberg. 1991. *Biomarkers*. New York: Simon & Schuster

CHAPTER 6

12 Hatfield, op.cit., 345

13 Institute of Medicine. 2012. *"Dietary Reference Intakes for Energy, Carbohydrates, Fiber, Fat, Fatty Acids, Cholesterol, Protein and Amino Acids."*: www.iom.edu

14 Berardi and Andrews, op. cit., 111-112

CHAPTER 8

15 Cleveland Clinic Journal of Medicine. 2013. *"Aspirin: its risks, benefits, and optimal use in preventing cardiovascular events."* www.cjm.org/content/80/5/318.full

17 Schaffer, S.W., and A.L. Harrison. 2007 "Aging of the Somatosensory System: A Translational Perspective." *Physical Therapy Journal.87:193-207.*

ABOUT THE AUTHOR

Master Fitness Trainer R.A.(Rich) Freedman is certified by the International Sports Sciences Association (ISSA). A graduate of Rutgers University in Economics, he retired from Shell Oil Company in 2000 after a 32 year career in business and finance having held a variety of management positions. He has been a registered commodities trader, Assistant General Auditor, and VP/ for several subsidiary companies as well as serving on their Board of Directors.

Rich was introduced to the world of professional training by former Washington Redskins' and Houston Texans' strength coach, Dan Riley. In 2003, he relocated to the Pacific Northwest where his wife finished out her career with the Portland Trail Blazers and he obtained further insight into professional sports training. In 2006, Rich received additional training under U.S. Olympic Coach, John Schaeffer, and received his ISSA certification. Since then Rich has also become an ISSA certified specialist in Fitness for Older Adults, Sports Nutrition, Exercise Therapy, Youth Fitness and Advanced Sports Conditioning. In November, 2011 Rich was awarded the title of "Master Trainer" by the ISSA. In May 2013, he became a Titleist Performance Institute (TPI) Certified Golf Fitness Instructor.

For the past 7 years Rich has trained both professional and amateur golfers at the Royal Oaks Country Club in Vancouver, WA. An author of several articles on health and wellness, he has served as a fitness consultant for the First Tee of Portland, OR and is currently on the Board of the Summit Golf Foundation which seeks to promote academic and life skills for children under state care in the Southwest Washington and Portland area. Rich also serves as the strength & conditioning coach for the Warner Pacific College Golf Team in Portland.

Rich and his wife Linda reside in Vancouver, WA and have 13 grandchildren.

CPSIA information can be obtained
at www.ICGtesting.com
Printed in the USA
FSOW03n0118061015
11865FS